Management and Professional Development for Nurses

Edited by

Mahrokh Dodwell

and

Judith Lathlean

Harper & Row, Publishers
London

Cambridge
Singapore
Philadelphia
New York

San Francisco
Mexico City
São Paulo
Sydney

Harper & Row Ltd
Middlesex House
34–42 Cleveland Street
London
W1P 5FB

British Library Cataloguing in Publication Data.

Management and professional development for nurses

1. Medicine – Nursing – Management
2. Dodwell, Mohrokh   II. Lathlean, Judith

610.73'068

ISBN: 0–06–318258–0

Typeset in 10/12pt Times Roman by Inforum Ltd, Portsmouth
Printed in Great Britain at the Alden Press, Oxford.

CONTENTS

List of contributors

Dee Borley Senior Officer, Royal College of Nursing, London.

Jane Burrows Regional Nurse (Planning), North Western Regional Health Authority, Manchester.

Robert Cooper Deputy Director of Nurse Education, Highland College of Nursing and Midwifery, Inverness.

Mahrokh Dodwell Formerly Project Director for the Postgraduate Teaching Hospitals' Sisters' Training Project, Royal Marsden Hospital, London.

Joanna Gray Consultant in Communication Skills, London.

Tom Kerrane Chief Nursing Officer and Quality Assurance Manager, National Heart and Chest Hospital, London.

Judith Lathlean Formerly Research Fellow, Nursing Research Unit, King's College, University of London. Now Independent Research Consultant in Nursing and Health Care, Peterborough.

Glynis Markham Director of Nursing Services, Royal Marsden Hospital, Sutton, Surrey.

Derek Reynolds Director of Finance and Information, Royal Marsden Hospital, London.

Foreword

The inadequacy of preparation for the role of the ward sister has been the subject of concern expressed regularly by the profession over the last two decades. Every major report on nursing education (Briggs, 1973; Judge, 1985; Project 2000, 1986) has identified the need to develop with some urgency management and professional education programmes for the ward sister. I welcome the publication of this book as it is a most timely addition to the literature on this subject.

The unique contribution that both the Editors have made in bringing together the 'fruits' of their teaching and research experience is to be commended. Although the book is based on one particular programme, its content has breadth and is practical in approach. The need to share experiences in the practice of education is important on two counts. Firstly we need to utilize limited and costly education resources more effectively, and secondly we need to improve evaluation techniques in order to enhance the quality of development programmes.

This book has an impressive range of contributors who have written with clarity on a number of complex subjects related to key components of the senior nurse's role. The concluding section on research and evaluation is a welcome inclusion as it is a critical subject that is often neglected. I believe the book will have wide appeal to students and to experienced registered nurses.

David Rye
Consultant in Nursing and Health Care

Preface

This is a book for all who care about continuing education and professional development, including those who consider that it is important for themselves and their staff, and those in education and management who are responsible for its promotion. The book by no means covers every issue and concern in continuing education as the field is far too broad. Rather we have selected aspects that we believe are currently causing concern, in the belief that they will stimulate ideas, raise questions and suggest avenues that readers may wish to explore further.

The idea for the book came originally from our experiences with the London Postgraduate Teaching Hospitals' programme for sisters. We are very grateful to this group of hospitals for the helpful and committed attitude of their staff, working with whom has been a pleasure. Many of the contributing authors have been associated with this programme. We are pleased that they have been able and willing to share their knowledge and expertise with a wider audience – the book has gained immeasurably from the vital part that they have played.

Although the plan for the book was originally developed by one of us (Mahrokh Dodwell) it soon became a collaborative arrangement with the inquisitive mind of a researcher challenging the ideas and experience of an educator and manager. This proved to be a rewarding partnership for both concerned.

Finally, we would like to thank Graham Dodwell and Robert Scott, our respective unfailing sources of support and confidence, who, as outsiders to the world of nursing and education, brought a much needed objective perspective.

Mahrokh Dodwell, London
Judith Lathlean, Peterborough

Introduction

Judith Lathlean and Mahrokh Dodwell

The context of nursing is changing, the demands increasing. And in the middle of this complexity is the sister or charge nurse, heralded as the 'lynchpin' of the service, the key to nursing standards, the focal point where the organization of nursing care and the needs of the patients meet. Yet research and studies have clearly shown that preparation and training for sisters are inadequate for their present roles let alone the future as envisaged by many of the statutory and professional nursing bodies. And further, the sister is often isolated, lacking in support, and bereft of the physical and emotional resources needed to do this demanding job.

The London Postgraduate Teaching Hospitals have attempted to remedy at least some of the deficiencies by establishing a programme for sisters which is 'creative, job related and flexible enough to meet the needs and complexities of this role, thus enabling individuals to contribute further to their organisation, enhance their future career prospects and promote excellence in nursing' (Dodwell and Lathlean, 1987). The idea for this book was conceived by the project director and was initiated by her desire to share the experiences of the programme with others. She in time joined forces with one of the evaluators of the programme, thus combining in the editorial a valuable external and internal perspective.

The editors make no apologies for setting the book in the context of one particular scheme. There is no one source of co-ordinated information about continuing professional education for nurses nor many published examples of how programmes have worked (or not) in practice. Learning takes place between managers, educators and practitioners by comparing notes and considering whether the experience of others matches or is appropriate for their own needs. This process of sharing avoids a costly re-inventing of the wheel whilst not purporting to offer a blueprint for success.

Although the book emanated from one particular innovation – and Chapter 2 provides an overview of this approach – the second part of the book has far broader implications and applicability. Each chapter tackles the fundamental issue of what senior practitioners (trained nurses but particularly sisters) need to know and do in order to function well and efficiently in clinical settings. The term 'ward sister' has been used most extensively but the relevance of the material is much wider and embraces departmental and specialty sisters and charge nurses in hospitals as well as the community nurse. For consistency, the feminine gender and the term 'sister' are used throughout to include both male and female sisters and charge nurses.

Research can help to improve practice and to monitor how well objectives are achieved throughout all aspects in nursing – practice, education and management. The final chapter, and third part of the book, considers both the relevance of research to nursing practice and the lessons that were learnt when a research approach was used to evaluate the programme. This provides a fitting conclusion to the book since it draws together the different elements discussed in the first two parts.

Professional development is a concern of all those working in the health service, both personally and in terms of the effect that well-prepared, trained and supported individuals have on the whole organization. It is a term used here to include everything that facilitates the extension and expansion of skills and knowledge which directly or indirectly result in improvements in personal and organizational performance, and ultimately contributes to higher standards of care provision. It is hoped that this book will therefore be of interest to those who care about their own development as well as those who have a responsibility for ensuring the development of others.

REFERENCE

Dodwell, M. and Lathlean, J. (1987) An innovative training programme for ward sisters, *Journal of Advanced Nursing*, Vol. 12, pp. 311–19.

Part One: The Context

1. Continuing Education: Option or Necessity?

Judith Lathlean and Mahrokh Dodwell

Change is inevitable. In a progressive country change is constant.

(Disraeli, 1867)

Despite a period of comparative stability in the 1950s and 1960s, the health service – and the nursing profession – has seen great and, in the past decade, constant change. This is the result of many influences from both outside and within the profession, and has led to quite different roles for the nurse practitioners of today. Education and professional development are vital factors both in the preparation of new entrants to the service and in enabling experienced individuals in nursing to fulfil their new and challenging roles.

Historically, nursing education has concentrated on preparation for entrance to one or more of the registers, for example, as a registered general nurse, registered mental nurse or enrolled nurse. For a minority of nurses this basic training has been supplemented by specialist, often clinical, courses (previously provided by the Joint Board and now the National Boards) and by very limited management training. So is there a need for more and different continuing education opportunities – or is it an optional extra that the service can ill afford? This chapter – and indeed the whole book – is aimed at demonstrating the importance of continuing professional education in the present context. It particularly focuses on sisters and charge nurses (the team leaders), since they have been acknowledged as the key group in nursing, but there are clear implications for all other levels of nurses from staff nurse through to managers.

THE CHANGING CONTEXT OF NURSING

The National Health Service has been in a state of flux and change since its inception in 1948 with a major reorganization in 1974, a Royal Commission in 1979 and, in the early 1980s, the introduction of general management as a result of a management inquiry – the Griffiths report (DHSS, 1983). Nursing in particular has been the subject of a number of reports affecting nursing management, for example, the Salmon report on senior nursing staff structure (Ministry of Health, 1966) and its community counterpart – the Mayston report (DHSS, 1969), and several relating to nursing education, for example, the Platt report (RCN, 1964), the Briggs report (DHSS, 1972), the Judge report (RCN, 1985), the English National Board's proposals (ENB, 1985) and Project 2000 (UKCC, 1986). In addition, there has been a recent green paper on primary health care, a report on community nursing (DHSS, 1986a) and a study of nursing skill mix (DHSS, 1986b). Thus the nursing profession has been bombarded with directives and recommendations which have changed its structure and in some ways the very nature of the profession.

Also, the context of nursing has altered – influenced by demographic, technological, political and economic factors. The scale of health-care provision is very different, systems have advanced and philosophies and values challenged. Clay (1987) points out that changes in the two ends of the population spectrum have dramatic effects on both the demand for services and the supply. In the demand for care, the number of elderly people – in particular the very elderly – is growing disproportionately. 'At present in NHS hospitals, almost 46 per cent of the acute beds are occupied by people over the age of 60' (Clay, 1987) and this figure is likely to increase during the next decade.

The second population change which affects the provision of health care is the sharp decline in the number of 18-year-olds from which nursing recruits.

In research especially undertaken for the RCN Commission for Nursing Education (RCN, 1985), it was found that by the early 1990s the drop in the number of suitably qualified young women school leavers with over five 'O' levels would be so great that nursing would need to take 50 per cent of that cohort just to maintain its current numbers. This target is clearly impossible.

(Clay, 1987)

Vigorous efforts are now being made not only to increase recruitment, but also to look at ways of retaining trained nurses in nursing.

The changing needs for health care and the manpower problems involved in providing that care are occurring alongside a greater interest in the health services by the consumer. The pressure for more consumer involvement in what is provided and how services are run grew during the 1970s resulting in the setting up of Community Health Councils. Interest at this level has also been matched by a gradually changing ethos at ward level with, for example, the emphasis on patient involvement in the planning of his care – a feature stressed by a nursing process approach to the organization of nursing care.

Nursing is affected as well by financial and economic factors. Between 1948 and the mid-1970s services expanded dramatically. However, the economic crisis in the 1970s brought an end to this major expansion and questions were raised about efficiency and effectiveness. This challenged the way whole groups were cared for; for example, the emphasis shifted from hospital to community care for the elderly, mentally ill and mentally handicapped. It also led to the abolition of a tier of health-service management in 1982 and 'competitive tendering' in 1983. The following two years saw the pursuit of 'efficiency savings' which the government were convinced could be made in the service.

The concept of cost-effectiveness is now important at ward level, particularly with the likelihood of limited – or no – expansion in services, and with the advent of devolved budgeting to wards and units. In addition, the efficiency of service provision, and the related administrative and support systems, has been the focus of attention. For example, patient administration systems (PAS) are being developed and performance indicators utilized. Some of these developments are dependent upon computer technology, highlighting another major change at ward level – the increased use of computers.

Parallel with attempts to become more efficient and cost-effective, the quality of care has been an important consideration. Both statutory and professional bodies, such as the DHSS and Royal College of Nursing, have promoted quality assurance – the measurement of the quality of care and the development of monitoring systems for quality control.

In summary, the context of nursing has changed considerably, the profession has been the subject of more scrutiny in recent years than hitherto, the expectations of the consumer have increased, resources have in some instances decreased, both efficiency and quality have been emphasized and the roles of many nurse practitioners have expanded and become more complex.

THE ROLE OF THE NURSE

Clearly these contextual and organizational changes have had a marked effect on the roles of nurses. So, for example, with advances in medicine and surgery, in some aspects nursing has also become more specialized. Moreover, hitherto unknown conditions such as AIDS raise technical, ethical and other issues for nursing. But perhaps the most fundamental issue – and the one that affects all trained nurses in whatever specialty – is that of accountability. This has received considerable emphasis from within the profession itself and matters related to it are likely to shape nursing in the foreseeable future.

The United Kingdom Central Council for Nurses, Midwives and Health Visitors has stated in the Code of Professional Conduct (UKCC, 1984) that 'each registered nurse, midwife and health visitor is account- able for his or her practice'. This statement is in line with the view of the Royal College of Nursing's Working Committee on Standards of Nursing Care who recommended that 'the professional accountability of the clinical nurse must be recognised' since 'accountability (being answerable for work and/or decisions about work) is the basis of professional standards' (RCN, 1981). They further suggest that good nursing care is achieved by the individual planning of care based on an assessment of individual needs, the systematic recording and subsequent review of the extent to which goals have been reached and the acceptance by each nurse of accountability for her individual nursing action. This approach to nursing (often referred to as the nursing process) has a direct bearing on the changing role of the nurse since this is not the way that many nurses have provided care in the past.

Most recently, there has been increasing support for primary nursing, that is

> a system for delivering nursing service that consists of four design elements: allocation and acceptance of individual responsibility for decision making to one individual; individual assignment of daily care; direct communica- tion channels; one person responsible for the quality of care administered to patients on a unit 24 hours a day, seven days a week.
>
> (Manthey, 1980)

This system not only affects the staff nurse who tends to be the primary nurse; it also changes the nature of the sister role in that she 'acts as a co-ordinator of nursing staff, a resource and information provider and a support giver' (Sparrow, 1986).

CONTINUING PROFESSIONAL EDUCATION

Continuing education has been described by the American Nurses' Association as 'planned educational activities intended to build upon the educational and experiential bases of the professional nurse for the enhancement of practice, education, administration, research or theory development to the end of improving the health of the public' (ANA, 1984). As such it encompasses post-basic education, in-service training and staff development programmes.

The need for continuing professional education

With changing roles has come the recognition that continuing education is essential. Basic nurse education can 'only be a foundation' (Royal Commission, 1979) but it should 'ensure a life-long progression of professional learning' (UKCC, 1986). The National Staff Committee (1981) stated that 'every nurse should be aware of the need to up-date and expand her knowledge and skills'. The Code of Conduct (UKCC, 1984) links this responsibility with the nurse's accountability.

In the exercise of professional accountability [the nurse] shall . . .

- Take every reasonable opportunity to maintain and improve professional knowledge and competence.
- Acknowledge any limitations of competence and refuse in such cases to accept delegated functions without first having received instruction in regard to those functions and having been assessed as competent.

In addition to the importance of continuing education for the up-dating and development of individuals, 'it is argued, and generally accepted, that an interested motivated workforce will perform more effectively than one which is neglected and disinterested' (Rogers and Lawrence, 1987). It is further suggested that continuing education opportunities can help to retain nurses in nursing (Lathlean, Smith and Bradley, 1986) and may attract former nurses back to practice.

The need for continuing education for nurses has been recognized for some years in North America where, it has been suggested, 'nurses demonstrate a considerable commitment to a great variety of continuing education' (Lahiff, 1984). The fact that the term 'continuing education' was defined by the American Nurses' Association in 1974, and subsequently revised in 1984, is an indication of the national view of its importance. In the United Kingdom although one professional group, the midwives, have had compulsory up-dating for some time, the nursing profession in general has been slow to respond. However, the principle of mandatory refreshment has now been established and the debate on how it should be done has begun (UKCC, 1987).

Other related initiatives are also happening, spurred on by the manpower crisis. For example, the NHS Management Board has set up a career development project group, aimed at examining career pathways for trained nurses and – significantly – their 'associated training and education needs'.

Participation in continuing education

A distinction tends to be made between post-basic education which leads to a nationally recognized qualification and in-service education for which there is no nationally recognized qualification. In respect of the former, a study was made of nurses undertaking Joint Board (now English National Board) post-basic clinical courses over the period 1973 to 1983 (Rogers, 1983). It was found that at the most only 9.7 per cent of qualified nurses could possess a post-basic clinical qualification and thus the opportunity for nurses to undertake these kinds of courses is very limited.

In a subsequent study by the same author – a survey of the opportunities for continuing professional education for nurses in health authorities – it was found that the provision made by different health districts was enormously variable and sometimes very sparse (Rogers and Lawrence, 1987). For example, the number of staff involved in delivering in-service and post-basic education ranged from 1 to 15 across the 175 districts who responded, less than half ran management courses, and only 2 per cent organized their own health-education courses.

Apart from the limited availability of places for continuing education events, time, motivation and lack of knowledge of opportunities are all factors affecting the involvement of nurses in continuing education. Also, in the past many nurses have been critical of management training, often organized off-site, because it appeared insufficiently related to their jobs. Even with the increase of in-service education and training there is still the feeling expressed by some that provision does not always reflect individual needs.

The changing concept of continuing education

Not only has the provision of continuing education for trained staff been limited, but also the concept has been fairly narrow. The tendency has been to equate it with courses and study days – formal provision made by the health authority that only restricted numbers of people can take part in. Rogers and Lawrence (1987) have also found that certain groups of nurses – notably enrolled nurses – feel particularly disadvantaged when it comes to the opportunity to participate in continuing education. Traditionally, part-time staff and night staff have also had problems of access.

Moreover, there has been criticism of the cost of involvement in such continuing education and whether the outcomes justify the expenditure. These factors pose a number of interrelated questions:

(1) How do people learn and what constitutes a 'learning opportunity'?
(2) How can better access to continuing education be achieved?
(3) Where does the responsibility for continuing education lie?
(4) What should be the focus of continuing education – the individual, the organization or both?

There are some indications that a broader notion of what constitutes continuing education is being developed within health districts although there is still considerable adherence to traditional views amongst both educators and potential participants. This is related to the first question – what constitutes a learning opportunity? And here the principles of adult learning are relevant. Knowles (1978) states that adults' orientation to learning is life-centred: therefore, it is more appropriate to study life or work situations rather than discrete subjects. Adults are motivated to learn as they experience needs that learning will satisfy. Moreover, they are self-directing in their learning and thus the role of the teacher is to engage in a process of mutual inquiry with them rather than transmit his or her knowledge to them and then evaluate their conformity to it. Almost a decade previously, Rogers (1969) stressed the importance of experience in considering that 'much significant learning is acquired through doing' and that 'learning is facilitated when the student participates responsibly in the learning process'.

Although such principles have been applied to methods of teaching in nursing for some years, though not always consistently, they have been slow to influence what is considered as an educational or development opportunity. Yet the potential for learning is enormous and the variety of ways in which this can take place is great. This is illustrated in Figure 1.1.

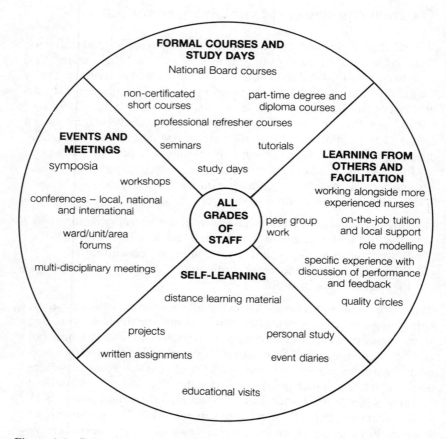

Figure 1.1 Potential opportunities for learning and continuing education

This wider vision of educational opportunities is also relevant to the question of availability of continuing education. Since learning and development occur in such a range of ways, although the availability of places on formalized courses and events may restrict access, all grades of staff can benefit from at least some of the opportunities. Further, this greater flexibility can allow the needs of individuals to be matched more closely with learning opportunities, a process which has been notoriously lacking in much continuing education and professional development.

There has also been a shift in view about the responsibility for continuing education. Hitherto, many have considered that this lies with the organization – that it has a duty to provide certain facilities for the employees who are merely passive recipients. However, there is now a move towards shared responsibility with more active involvement of individuals in identifying their needs and ways of meeting those needs. This has been facilitated by the expansion of distance learning and other methods which are essentially self-directed and is made more feasible by the greater range of possibilities, many of which are far less costly and viable.

In the past continuing education has been very much focused on individuals. Often isolated people have taken part in a multitude of disparate courses and events with hopefully personal gain but limited chance of effecting change in the organization. Rogers and Lawrence's (1987) study found that only 58 per cent of Districts claimed to have a specific philosophy for continuing education and 41 per cent claimed specific policies. The absence in so many instances of an overall plan is a significant factor in the haphazard pattern of continuing education.

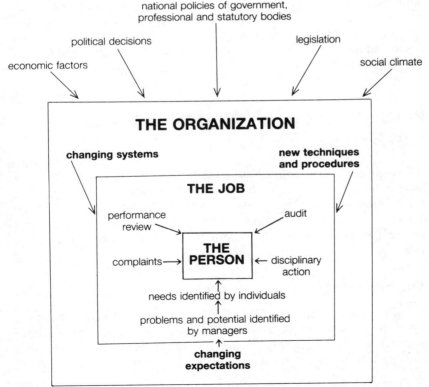

Figure 1.2 Factors influencing both organizational and staff development

However, the need to balance organizational requirements with individual needs is becoming increasingly recognized particularly since the former have become so critical; for example, the organization's need to retain nurses in nursing and tackle the manpower wastage, the severe problems of recruitment, the concerns over standards of care, and the emphasis on cost-effectiveness and measurement of performance. To this end, Lathlean, Smith and Bradley (1986) recommended that 'each district should identify a particular officer who has lead responsibility for the development of individuals and the organisation', a proposition that has received the support of the English National Board's Continuing Education Committee.

The interrelationship between the organization, the job and the individual, and the factors giving rise to the need for both organizational and individual development are illustrated in Figure 1.2.

Concepts of continuing education change slowly and it will be a long time before comprehensive programmes are developed in all health authorities. Also, organizations have their own priorities and, when resources are limited, the decision of many organizations is to start first with priority areas and build upon them. In this respect, many would argue that the starting point in continuing nurse education should be the development of the sister role.

PROFESSIONAL DEVELOPMENT FOR SISTERS

Although continuing education and development are important at all levels, the role that can probably reap most benefits from increased preparation and training – both in terms of the organization and the individual – is that of the sister since she is 'the only nurse who has direct managerial responsibilities for both patients and nurses' (Pembrey, 1980).

The importance of the sister role

Studies related to the role of the sister are not new – descriptions of the sister as a manager and teacher date back to the era of Florence Nightingale. More recently, in the late 1950s, Menzies – in her well known study of stress in nursing (Menzies, 1960) – argued that sisters are deprived of potential satisfaction in their roles because many of them would like closer contact with their patients, but are prevented from having this because of the demands of teaching students.

The *teaching* role of the sister has been highlighted by many researchers in the late 1970s and early 1980s (see, for example, Orton, 1981; Fretwell, 1982; Marson, 1982 and Ogier, 1982.) The message coming clearly from the research was the importance of the sister in setting the 'tone' of the ward as an effective 'learning environment' and the difficulties that many sisters experienced in finding the time to teach, exacerbated by their lack of confidence and preparation (Farnish, 1983).

Other research studies have concentrated on the importance of the sister in controlling the *communication* flow into and within the ward (Lelean, 1973) and the *management* function of the sister. Pembrey (1980) identified the sister as 'the key nurse in negotiating the care of the patient because she is the only person in the nursing structure who actually and symbolically represents continuity of care for the patient'. Further, it tends to be the sister who sets the standards of care (RCN, 1980). In addition, the fact that the sister acts as a 'role model', facilitating the learning for her ward staff, has also been stressed (Pembrey, 1980; Runciman, 1983). There is clearly not just one effective way of managing a ward although certain features of 'good' role models have been described such as enthusiasm and high motivation and loyalty to the nursing team.

Thus the role of the ward sister has been the focus of many research studies and attention from committees, statutory and professional bodies, particularly in the past decade. They all refer to the importance and complexity of the role; quite a number are concerned with the inability of many sisters to fulfil their 'full' role, for example, the teaching or the managerial aspects. Various reasons are given for the deficiencies such as lack of skill and preparation, different priorities and views about the role, lack of time, shortage of staff and the need for support. Solutions are offered such as more preparation and development opportunities, encouragement to organize the role in alternative ways, and the provision of support. The sister's lack of preparation for – and training within – her role has emerged strongly from several of these studies, particularly those of Pembrey (1980), Farnish (1983) and Lathlean and Farnish (1984).

Recently, the message of these studies has been reinforced by an unequivocal statement from the Chief Executive of the NHS Management Board, made to all regional general managers. He strongly recommended that in view of the crucial importance of the leader of the ward nursing team in maximising the quality and cost-effectiveness of patient care, authorities should make every effort to provide the necessary training and management, financial and analytical support to facilitate the work of ward sisters and charge nurses.

(DHSS, 1986c)

THE WAY FORWARD

The message is clear. If nurses are to cope with the ever increasing demands on the service both for greater provision and for more effective ways of achieving good patient care then they require the requisite skills and knowledge as well as the resources to do the job. A vital way of ensuring adequate skills and knowledge is by a systematic, planned yet flexible programme of professional development and learning opportunities. The benefits of this can be considerable and reach far beyond the individual nurse, influencing such important issues as the likelihood of nurses staying or leaving in clinical nursing, the level of morale in practice settings and the standards of nursing care achieved.

This has to be a concern of the general manager since he is ultimately accountable for the maximization of resources in the best interests of both the staff employed by the authority and the service provided for patients. Where professional and organizational development are concerned, though statutory and professional bodies may define policies and provide guidelines, ultimately it is the initiatives in the health districts that are likely to have the greatest impact on local standards and performance. Chapter 2 illustrates possibilities by giving some insight into one particular approach – a strategy that can be adapted and used in many other settings and for other grades of staff.

REFERENCES

American Nurses' Association (1984) *Standards for Continuing Education in Nursing*, American Nurses' Association, Missouri.
Clay, T. (1987) *Nurses: Power and Politics*, Heinemann, London.
Department of Health and Social Security (1969) *Report of the Working Party on Management Structure in the Local Authority Nursing Services*, Chairman, E.C. Mayston, HMSO, London.
Department of Health and Social Security (1972) *Report of the Committee on Nursing* (Briggs Report), HMSO, London.

Department of Health and Social Security (1983) *NHS Management Inquiry Report* (Griffiths Report), HMSO, London.
Department of Health and Social Security (1986a) *Neighbourhood Nursing: A Focus for Care* (Cumberlege Report), HMSO, London.
Department of Health and Social Security (1986b) *Mix and Match: A Review of Nursing Skill Mix*, DHSS, London.
Department of Health and Social Security (1986c) *Memorandum to Regional General Managers on Nursing Manpower*, 13 June.
Disraeli, B. (1867) From *Speech at Edinburgh*, 19 October 1867.
English National Board for Nursing, Midwifery and Health Visiting (1985) *Professional Education/Training Courses: Consultation Paper*, ENB, London.
Farnish, S. (1983) *Ward Sister Preparation: A Survey in Three Districts*, NERU Report No. 2, Nursing Education Research Unit, Chelsea College, University of London.
Fretwell, J. (1982) *Ward Teaching and Learning*, Royal College of Nursing, London.
Knowles, M. (1978) *The Adult Learner: A Neglected Species*, Gulf Publishing Co., Houston.
Lahiff, M. (1984) 'A step further' in King's Fund Centre, *Continuing Education in Nursing – Luxury or Necessity*, Report of a Conference, King Edward's Hospital Fund for London.
Lathlean, J. and Farnish, S. (1984) *The Ward Sister Training Project: An Evaluation of a Training Scheme*, NERU Report no. 3, Chelsea College, University of London.
Lathlean, J., Smith, G. and Bradley, S. (1986) *Post-Registration Development Schemes Evaluation*, NERU Report no. 4, King's College, University of London.
Lelean, S. (1973) *Ready for Report, Nurse?* Royal College of Nursing, London.
Manthey, M. (1980) *The Practice of Primary Nursing*, Blackwell, Oxford.
Marson, S. (1982) Ward sister – teacher or facilitator? An investigation into the behavioural characteristics of effective ward teachers, *Journal of Advanced Nursing*, Vol. 7, pp. 347–57.
Menzies, I.E.P. (1960) A case study in the functioning of social systems as a defence against anxiety, *Human Relations*, Vol.13, no.2, pp. 95–121.
Ministry of Health, Scottish Home and Health Department (1966) *Report of the Committee on Senior Nursing Staff Structure*, Chairman, B. Salmon, HMSO, London.
National Staff Committee for Nurses and Midwives (1981) *Recommendations on the Organisation and Provision of Continuing In-service Education and Training*, DHSS, London.
Ogier, M. (1982) *An Ideal Sister?* Royal College of Nursing, London.
Orton, H. (1981) Ward learning climate and student nurse response, *Nursing Times Occasional Paper*, Vol.77, no.17, pp. 65–8.
Pembrey, S.E.M. (1980) *The Ward Sister: Key to Nursing*, Royal College of Nursing, London.
Rogers, C. (1969) *Freedom to Learn*, C.N. Merril, Columbus, Ohio.
Rogers, J. (1983) *The Follow Up Study of the Careers of Nurses Who Had Completed a JBCNS Certificate Course*, DHSS, London.
Rogers, J. and Lawrence, J. (1987) *Continuing Professional Education for*

Qualified Nurses, Midwives and Health Visitors, Ashdale Press, Peterborough.

Royal College of Nursing (1964) *A Reform of Nursing Education*, Chairman, Platt, RCN, London.

Royal College of Nursing (1980) *Standards of Nursing Care*, Royal College of Nursing, London.

Royal College of Nursing (1981) *Towards Standards*, Royal College of Nursing, London.

Royal College of Nursing (1985) *The Education of Nurses: A New Dispensation*, Chairman, Judge, Royal College of Nursing, London.

Royal Commission on NHS (1979) HMSO, London.

Runciman, P. (1983) *Ward Sister at Work*, Churchill Livingstone, Edinburgh.

Sparrow, S. (1986) Primary nursing, *Nursing Practice*, Vol. 1, pp. 142–8.

United Kingdom Central Council for Nursing, Midwifery and Health Visitors (1984) *Code of Professional Conduct*, UKCC, London.

United Kingdom Central Council for Nursing, Midwifery and Health Visitors (1986) *Project 2000: A New Preparation for Practice*, UKCC, London.

United Kingdom Central Council for Nursing, Midwifery and Health Visitors (1987) *Mandatory Periodic Refreshment for Nurses and Health Visitors*. Discussion Paper, UKCC, London.

2. A Training Programme for Sisters

Mahrokh Dodwell

PREPARATION AND TRAINING FOR SISTERS

> The role outlined for the sister implies extensive clinical expertise and a preparation for clinical management in excess of the present provision.
>
> (RCN, 1981)

Specific training for sisters has been slow to develop despite the acknowledged importance of the role. Following the Salmon report in the mid-1960s (Ministry of Health, 1966), first-line management training for nurses was promoted. However, it was estimated in 1968 that 33,000 sisters needed to be considered for management training and that the annual number of places required would be 4,300. Understandably, provision did not keep pace with need. Also, there were problems in mounting a large-scale system of training. Williams studied the role of the ward sister (Williams, 1969) and looked at the analysis of training needs. He stressed that all hospitals would have different needs and that in the design of training programmes, there must be sufficient flexibility for local considerations to be taken into account.

Evaluation of first-line management courses on a national basis appeared lacking but some local studies indicated that although staff who attended courses generally enjoyed them they had difficulty in applying the knowledge gained to their jobs. Farnish (1983) found that some sisters referred to their experiences as 'the sheep-dip approach' or 'the conveyor belt'. 'There was little apparent relationship between theory and practice (in the ward situation) and sisters were alienated by the emphasis on the academic and industry-orientated approach to management' (Lathlean and Farnish, 1984).

Davies (1972) undertook a detailed evaluation of first-line management courses for newly appointed ward sisters in the Manchester Region, between 1968 and 1970. She found that there were certain factors which appeared to inhibit the achievement of the course objectives including:

- the physical distance of the course members from their organizational realities (the hospitals);
- the gap between the lecturers, who lacked hospital experience and relied on conceptual teaching, and the course members, whose previous training was mainly of a practical nature;
- the difference in the value systems of the two groups, with the industrial concepts of profit and the economic use of resources being viewed by course members as irrelevant to their professional system of values.

In summary,

> existing courses were seen as ineffective because they 'concentrate on changing the individual' who has difficulty in initiating change; they are run outside the hospitals and do not involve the senior staff; there are many pressures in a ward situation which 'encourage a sister to return to her pre-course behaviour pattern'; they 'challenge some of the basic assumptions of the organisational structure and question the patient-orientated value system of the nurse'.

> (Lathlean and Farnish, 1984)

Interestingly, although there has been some change in attitudes and philosophy, for example, an increased emphasis in nursing on the economic use of resources and a greater acceptance of the relevance of knowledge and theory from outside the profession, many of these concerns are just as relevant today as they were nearly twenty years ago.

By the late 1970s, there was a considerable unease about the appropriateness of first-line management courses. Concern was related to their apparent ineffectiveness, costliness, discrepancy between availability and demand, and their often poor timing for the individuals involved (Redfern, 1981). Some hospitals started their own management courses to remedy these deficiencies. Nevertheless, many of these remained relatively unrelated to the roles of the course members, relied on teaching methods which were essentially didactic rather than experiential, were focused on global topics instead of taking account of the needs of individuals and were often directed towards current practices rather than developing the potential of participants.

However, a firm move away from this pattern was pioneered in 1979 by the establishment of an experimental training scheme for ward sisters, supported by the King Edward's Hospital Fund for London (King's Fund). The scheme was run in two hospitals and was evaluated over a three-and-a-half year period. (A report of this evaluation is available – Lathlean and Farnish, 1984.) The scheme was based on four premises: there is a need for specific training for ward sisters; this training should be ward-based; it requires a joint education/service approach; and nurses learn how to become sisters by observing the behaviour of other, more experienced ward sisters.

It was suggested that 'the best and quickest method for preparation of ward sisters is in the real life situation: where the nurse will encounter the day-to-day problems of running a ward, but will have the advantage of the support of a tutor to guide her studies and an experienced ward sister to act as a role model' (Davies, 1981). Thus the course members (trainees) spent three months in a designated training ward run by an experienced ward sister (known as a sister preceptor) with a nurse tutor primarily responsible for organizing the theoretical input of the course, and for providing support for the trainees. 'During the second three months, the ward sister trainee takes up appointment in her ward and is supported and observed not only by her nursing officer but also by the tutor/preceptor' (Wood, 1982).

The overall aim of the course was to prepare registered general nurses to function efficiently as ward sisters in the areas of their role relating to: the management of patient care, teaching, ward management, personnel management and nursing research. It was expected that learning would take place in a variety of ways: through shadowing the ward sister preceptor (the role model) and critically discussing and analysing her performance; by seminars, tutorials and discussions on aspects of the sister's work; by visits to other institutions and departments; by written assignments and by critical feedback on performance during the second three months.

The evaluation found that there were considerable developments in the participants but did highlight a number of constraints and problems with this type of scheme. For example, it proved to be very stressful for one ward sister preceptor to act as the role model for the trainees particularly when the numbers increased from two per course to four or five. There was also the consideration of 'overload' with the large number of supernumerary course members, whose roles were rather uncertain, being on the ward at the same time. Further, although the first part of the course seemed 'just about the right length' for most or 'only marginally too long' for others, the second three months barely felt to be an integral part of the programme for the majority, and their needs for contact, input and support varied greatly during this time.

The evaluation project concluded that the sister role was indeed a crucial one. It reinforced the need for specific investment in the preparation and training of sisters, the value of looking critically at the role in different settings, the merit of organizing the experience of sisters to maximize the learning that takes place from observing other sisters, and the need of sisters (particularly when newly appointed) for support in developing their own practice.

The options to be considered include the focus of the training – should it be for the sister when just appointed to her first post or when she is slightly more experienced, or maybe it is better to train the senior staff nurse when she is ready to apply for a sister's post? The location of the programme is another consideration; schemes based in one hospital – or even one district – may suffer from a lack of potential candidates but more widely based schemes, such as regional, can lack identity with the person's workplace. Also, the best structure for the programme is debatable. Although 'there appears to be merit in a programme with two aspects – one concentrating on the more formal elements of learning and the other on the application of this learning in a supportive environment – this can be organised in a number of different ways' (Lathlean and Farnish, 1984) such as a programme with separate modules between which the participant returns to her workplace. Also, whilst the King's Fund scheme was of fixed duration, an alternative could be planned which is more flexible, open-ended and individually tailored.

A PROGRAMME FOR THE POSTGRADUATE TEACHING HOSPITALS

In the early 1980s, although several health authorities were beginning to develop their training and education opportunities for sisters, there were few reported programmes apart from the King's Fund scheme and another role-based programme in the Oxfordshire Health Authority. Awareness of the key position occupied by the sister encouraged the London Postgraduate Teaching Hospitals' Joint Education and Training Committee (representing seven hospitals) to hold a nursing conference on the subject in August 1982. As a result, 'ways in which the role of the ward sister could be developed within the postgraduate teaching hospitals were examined in relation to current practice and studies that had been carried out on the role of the ward sister' (Dodwell and Lathlean, 1987). The existing schemes were studied to help decide upon the best way forward for the Postgraduate Teaching Hospitals. Consequently certain principles and aspects of the King's Fund scheme were thought to be appropriate, particularly the structure and content of the curriculum, the emphasis on role modelling, the use of facilitators to assist in the learning and the involvement of an independent evaluator. But the Postgraduate Teaching Hospitals were keen to set up a programme that met their own needs and therefore used the experience of others as a guide rather than a prescription.

The reasons for including a fairly detailed description of the programme are various and were raised in the Introduction to this book. It should be stressed, though, that it is not presented as a blueprint for action but more an illustration of an approach that might provide guidance for others and a basis for comparison with alternatives.

The establishment of the programme

The setting up of the programme was an innovative process since few precedents existed, and no programmes were identified that exactly matched the requirements of the seven hospitals comprising the London Postgraduate Teaching Hospitals group. The programme was based on a number of principles and evaluated throughout an initial experimental period. The planning, whilst initiated by a project director, was a collaborative venture with all seven hospitals involved.

The basis for the programme
A number of principles influenced the planning and design of the programme including:

- the appropriateness of getting individuals to identify their own particular needs, strengths and weaknesses;
- the importance of involving managers in the assessment process – both of needs and performance;
- the value of the facilitator role to act as a link between education and service and provide support in the translation of theory into practice;
- the importance of a co-ordinator whose role is not only to organize and develop the programme but also to provide support for participants (course members) and facilitators;
- the need not only to concentrate on the current role but also to prepare for the future;

- the need to recognize participants as adult learners and use methods suitable for them.

Staff and structure

The key person in the development and progress of the programme was the project director, a person with a combined clinical, management and education background, appointed to the project in May 1983. Her main role initially was to plan and organize the programme, liaise with the seven participating hospitals, and set up a system for the selection of participants. Apart from the involvement of the chief nursing officer for each hospital, facilitators were nominated from both service and education positions. (The role of these facilitators is described in more detail later in the chapter.)

The programme was based on a modular system with week-long study blocks interspersed with ward placements, preferably in a different ward from the course members' own. A further optional period of two weeks was planned for additional study and activities with a one-day follow up for the whole programme. Emphasis was placed on a variety of methods being used in the study weeks, particularly those encouraging maximum participation of participants.

Aims and objectives

The programme was aimed at preparing registered general nurses to function effectively and efficiently in the role as ward sister. The overall objectives of the programme were to assist sisters:

- to apply management principles to their work environment;
- to understand their organizational role in communication and the co-ordination of the resources;
- to analyse their leadership and management style and seek ways for improvement through effective performance review and career planning.

The role was considered to have five elements: clinical management, ward management, personnel management, teaching and learning, and research, and detailed objectives for the course were centred around these five topics (see Figure 2.1).

Planning and monitoring

The responsibility for the planning of the programme lay in the main with the project director but the chief nursing officers of all seven hospitals, together with the project director, formed a planning committee. This group met every few months throughout the experimental period to discuss major matters in relation to the programme including the objectives, the curriculum, the appointment and use of facilitators, selection to the programme and the evaluation. A particular concern of the senior managers was to identify the corporate needs of their hospitals that could be met or at least ameliorated by the further education and development of their nursing staff at sister level.

Issues of principle rather than detail were debated in this forum. For example, to what extent should the programme aim to be remedial or should the emphasis be more on future development of the role? Initially views about, and commitment to, the programme were not consistent throughout the group and the meetings gave a focus to discussions about purpose, process and outcome.

Few innovative experimental programmes are set up nowadays without some method of evaluation – and this scheme was no exception. Initially it was hoped that an independent evaluation would be undertaken throughout the whole experimental period by an external researcher working in collaboration with the project director. Unfortunately, since no funding was forthcoming, after the system for evaluation had been set up the role of the external researcher had to be reduced to an advisory one, the main responsibility for evaluation falling to the project director. The project director was supported in this activity by the director of research of one of the hospitals. (The evaluation methods are described in Chapter 10.) The outcomes of the evaluation were fed back to the chief nursing officers and the facilitators, thus allowing discussion and decisions about necessary modifications to the programme.

Ascertaining learning needs

Nurses should be involved in the assessment of their own needs and the needs of individuals for education and development should be considered together with those of the organization (Lathlean, Smith and Bradley, 1986; Rogers and Lawrence, 1987). These principles influenced the process that was adopted in both designing the programme and in finding out who could most benefit from it and how.

The curriculum was developed by extensive reference to research and other sources indicating the nature of the sister role, the relationship of the role to the nursing team and the wider context, the problems, constraints and challenges. Account was also taken of national directives (though few existed), policies and priorities. It was then debated with the

CLINICAL MANAGEMENT

Objectives

The nurse will be able to:
- Discuss the philosophy of nursing and identify principles of clinical nursing management.
- Discuss the role and responsibility of the ward sister in the delivery of patient care.
- Describe the sister's role in monitoring and maintaining high standards of care.
- Describe the techniques she may use to assess needs, plan care, implement and develop tools for evaluating care for a patient/group of patients.
- Demonstrate ability to maintain accurate written records.
- Discuss ethical and legal implications in the treatment and care of patients in her area.

WARD MANAGEMENT

Objectives

The nurse will be able to:
- Demonstrate the ability to act as team leader.
- Identify needs of patients/relatives.
- Identify priorities.
- Identify and utilize resources available.
- Delegate responsibility within the team.
- Communicate with patients/relatives/ward staff and other members of health-care team and promote good working relationships.
- Identify work problems and acquire a systematic approach to problem solving and decision making.
- Plan effective duty and holiday rotas.
- Discuss the procedures for
    Staff grievance,
    Complaints.
- Define leadership and identify the various leadership styles.
- Demonstrate efficient ward organization and economical use of resources.
- Evaluate ward management and plan short- and long-term goals.
- Identify staff support systems available.
- Recognize her responsibilities in providing a safe environment.
- Identify the structure and function of Health Service provision.
- Describe the structure of professional organizations.

PERSONNEL MANAGEMENT

Objectives

The nurse will be able to:
- Identify the role of the ward sister in personnel management.
- Identify the need for professional development.
- Participate in her own staff development and performance review.
- Show an awareness of the importance of industrial relations.
- Identify the need for staff welfare and be aware of the available facilities.
- Promote high morale amongst staff.

- Identify the role of the senior nurse managers and other health care professionals.
- Recognize effects of stress on staff and self and to identify how it can be averted.
- Recognize the need for counselling.
- Outline the skills for effective counselling.

TEACHING AND LEARNING

Objectives

The nurse will be able to:
- Discuss the learning needs of
  Junior staff,
  Patients and relatives.
- Discuss factors which either promote or hinder learning.
- Describe teaching methods and aids.
- Demonstrate the ability to teach patients, relatives, learners and other staff.
- Identify, select, prepare and use relevant teaching methods.
- Assess learners' progress and performance.
- Discuss and advise learners about their performance and write a report at the end of the review.

RESEARCH

Objectives

The nurse will be able to:
- Discuss the relationship of research to nursing.
- Describe the research process.
- Critically analyse research findings.
- Describe how research findings can apply to clinical practice.
- Encourage research awareness in other nursing staff.
- Recognize ethical aspects of research involving nurses and patients.

Figure 2.1 The curriculum

senior managers to ensure a good fit between individual needs and those of the constituent hospitals. It was during this stage, for example, that the managers endorsed the need for a substantial input about research and teaching since skills and knowledge in these areas were considered to 'require improvement'.

Needs identification was also part of the procedure established for selecting and preparing participants for the programme. Selection for the course was based on the apparent ability of individuals to benefit from it, either because they were newly appointed to the post, since it is known that sisters benefit from additional input and support at this time, or because they had received little or no previous preparation or training for their sister role or, in the case of staff nurses, they showed potential for promotion to a sister's post.

Facilitators met with prospective course members prior to their attendance on the first module – often in conjunction with the nurse's manager – in order to find out in what areas of the role the participant needed help. This information could then be relayed to the project director who could use it to ensure that various topics were covered and also to offer additional support to individuals if necessary. Special needs could sometimes be catered for in the programme but were often taken up in the optional two-week period of the course. The recording of the information about individual needs formed part of the evaluation and assessment process.

Designing the programme

The design of the programme was based on the tried and tested experience of others involved in the training and development of sisters and on the particular needs of the organizations and individuals, informed by knowledge of how adults best learn. Through the evaluation and experience of the earlier courses, the contents and methods used were to be modified. A complex network of influences was relevant in the development of the programme – the thoughts, experiences and assessments of the course members, the views of the facilitators and managers, changes in the organizations giving rise to different needs and contingencies, national pressures and priorities – but the co-ordinator of all the activity at the grass roots remained the project director.

Resources

'If managers believe that the ward sister role is crucial in ensuring effective clinical management . . . then they will be prepared to allocate resources for specific training' (Lathlean and Farnish, 1984). A criticism of continuing education has been the tendency for some authorities to provide isolated and fragmented opportunities such as odd study days and events which do not form part of a coherent whole and are attended by individuals in a random and *ad hoc* way. The reasons are often financial and sometimes an indication of a 'lip-service' approach to continuing education. Yet it is known that such arrangements are often far from cost effective since there is only likely to be a limited increase in knowledge and skills and virtually no lasting professional development from attendance at a one-day event with no preparation, matching to needs or follow up.

Therefore, a programme of this kind does require commitment to the allocation of resources – a commitment that the group of hospitals was in agreement about making. The main financial implication was the appointment of a project director for a three-year period. This feature, however, appears to be *fundamental* to the success of a programme and is cost-effective since the role combines many activities – programme planning and implementation, liaison between managers, course members and others involved with the programme, support for participants, and evaluation and programme development. Without co-ordination which spans education and service such an innovation can flounder.

Other resource implications include the cost of participants being away from their wards or units for four weeks (and more if the optional two weeks are taken up); the cost of replacing the nurse whilst away (if this is done); the resources of the school; fees of outside lecturers; secretarial time and stationery, and other incidentals. An actual financial assessment would also need to take into consideration the time facilitators and managers spend with course members, attending meetings related to the programme and completing assessment and evaluation forms in respect of individuals involved. However, it could be argued that aspects of this (such as discussing with nurses their needs and performance) should in any case be part of the role of the manager and therefore not counted as a separate cost.

THE PROGRAMME IN ACTION

The course is spread over six months and comprises four separate study blocks of one week each, with three placements of approximately three weeks each between blocks. There are two weeks for additional study and visits to other units within or outside the hospital, but often this option

Study blocks and placements	Duration
Introductory block	1 week
Placement	3 weeks approx.
Block 2	1 week
Placement	3 weeks approx.
Block 3	1 week
Placement	3 weeks approx.
Final block	1 week
Optional additional study	2 weeks
Follow-up day	1 day

Figure 2.2   Structure of the programme

has not been taken up. A follow-up day for feedback and presentation of certificates takes place at the end of the six months (see Figure 2.2)

Participants

The programme was initially specifically aimed at the newly appointed sister in general and specialist wards and areas. As a result of the early evaluation the emphasis on inexperienced sisters was reinforced but the programme was also considered to be of value to more experienced sisters and senior staff nurses. Thus although the newly appointed sisters have priority for places other trained nurses benefit too from the programme.

Each course takes a maximum of approximately twenty participants, the majority being sisters with less than one year's experience, from a variety of general and specialist settings including midwifery, paediatrics, psychiatry, night duty, outpatients, theatres and community nursing. Course members are selected by the chief nursing officers of each of the Postgraduate Teaching Hospitals, the aim being to have a mix of participants from across the seven hospitals.

Course content and curriculum

The course attempts to cover the areas of the sister role as comprehensively as possible, as well as include the opportunity for sisters from different wards and specialties to pursue topics of particular relevance to themselves. Subjects include those which affect the context of nursing as well as those which impinge directly upon the role of the sister. They attempt to consolidate existing knowledge, experience and skills in clinical issues, management, interpersonal skills, research, law, professional awareness and development and the like as well as expand upon these areas.

'Clinical nursing management' is concerned with the role of the sister in the daily management of patient care. Consideration is made of the use of different models of nursing and approaches which involve assessing patients, needs, planning care, implementing and evaluating care. Strategies for monitoring care and ensuring high standards of care (including quality assurance) are focused upon since it is known from research that it is the sister who determines the quality of care provided in clinical settings. The legal and ethical implications of managing care are also included, as is the importance of maintaining accurate records. 'Ward management' considers the responsibilities of the sister as a manager, both her relationship to and role within the wider context of policies, planning and resource management and to her ward or unit. The former includes the part played by sisters in the management of financial resources (Chapter 3), particularly in the light of moves towards devolved budgeting to ward/unit level, her role in the management of manpower – an increasingly critical issue for nursing – and the relationship of the sister to the planning process (Chapter 4).

The programme also explores her role in the ward or unit as a leader, and the qualities of leadership and leadership styles. It is known that sisters are key people in the control and co-ordination of information in the ward, both with patients and staff (Lelean, 1973) and therefore emphasis is placed on this topic including the analysis of factors hindering and helping effective communication (Chapter 6).

A problem-solving approach with a systematic cycle of identification of issues, planning, implementation and evaluation is the basis for many of the aspects of ward management. The role of the sister in the management of change and in coping with uncertainty is also highlighted since her ability to perform within an 'organic', dynamic organization and, at the same time facilitate change, is increasingly vital in nursing at ward level. With the greater pressures in wards and units the staff tend to expect the sister as team leader to take the initiative both in terms of patient care and in the management of the ward staff.

'Personnel management' includes a range of functions such as the sister's role in staff appraisal and performance review, a subject which is included in some depth in the programme (Chapter 5), the promotion of morale in a ward/unit setting, knowledge and skills in industrial relations (Chapter 8), the recognition of stress in the nursing team and in herself, the skills of effective counselling and the identification of needs in her staff for support (Chapter 9). Assertiveness training is an aspect of this topic and peer review is also included. The importance of the sister's involvement in interviewing and selecting staff is reinforced since if, as a manager, she is to be accountable for the work of others she should be in a position of influence as to who her staff are to be.

'Teaching and learning' involves the identification of needs amongst ward nurses, patients and their relatives, the development of teaching skills and the assessment of progress and performance (Chapter 7).

'Research' is concerned more with the appreciation of research and the use of research findings to improve clinical practice, rather than the

	Monday	Tuesday	Wednesday	Thursday	Friday
Week 1	Introduction and orientation to course; History of nursing management; Principles of management	Financial management; Tips on audio-visual aids; Importance of clinical nursing management; Accountability	Management of change workshop; Library visit	Counselling and interpersonal skills workshop (All day)	Leadership workshop • team building • motivation • styles of leadership; Communication • principles • methods • tools
Week 2	Teaching and learning • theories and methods • using the environment • learning needs • factors that promote Leadership • decision-making • delegation	Future nursing structure; Employment law and contract of employment; Nursing models; Nursing process	The nurse and the law; Practical responsibilities of the sister; Teaching and learning • theories and methods of teaching • setting objectives	Nursing research • research methods • relevance to nursing; Disciplinary and grievance procedure (Video: I'd like a word with you); Nursing process	Role of the nurse in health education; NHS structure and future; Nursing research • ethical and legal issues; Service planning • effective use of resources
Week 3	Standards of care; Staff appraisal and performance review (Video: How am I doing?); Future of nurse education; Capital planning	Committee skills (Agenda, minutes, report writing); Health and safety at work (and video); Bereavement • grief process • coping	Professional and statutory bodies in nursing; Therapeutic development; Management of aggression and violence	Nursing research • the application of findings to clinical practice; Application of performance indicators; Workshop: 'stress coping'	Nursing research • product evaluation; Politics of health care; Workshop: writing for publication; Assertiveness training
Week 4	Workshop: Evaluation of care • Quality assurance; Role of the General Manager; Public image of the nurse	International nursing; Communication • written • factors that hinder and promote; Use of computers in nursing	The nurse and the law; Management of time; Nursing ethics; Group discussion and problem-solving exercises	Interviewing skills and video; Dealing with complaints; The role of the CHC; Counselling • staff support	Presentation of case history/research review (Microteaching/video feedback); Evaluation of the course

Figure 2.3   Sample four-week programme

undertaking of a research study (Chapter 10).

A typical programme for the four week-long blocks is shown in Figure 2.3. Each programme varies slightly according to the needs of the participants in that programme, the feedback from the evaluation of previous programmes, and with the presenters of the individual topics.

Methods

A variety of teaching methods is used including lectures, seminars, workshops, self-directed and experiential methods with greater emphasis on participative rather than didactic approaches. These are supported by audio-visual aids, films, video feedback and role play. Wherever possible, course members are encouraged to accept a shared responsibility for learning – hence the orientation towards involvement in the learning opportunity, with the tutor or 'specialist' acting as facilitator rather than teacher.

The speakers for each programme are from within and outside the Postgraduate Teaching Hospitals which has the advantage of involving staff who are part of the constituent hospitals in the training of their own sisters and external 'specialists' who can bring a wider, sometimes national perspective.

Participants are expected to complete a number of written assignments. For example, a short essay on the 'Role of the ward sister' is prepared at the beginning and at the end of the course to help identify course members' views and knowledge at the start and highlight changes in their perceptions after participation in the programme. In addition, they prepare and present to the group a teaching aid of their choice, a nursing care/case study and a critical review of a research report or a small research project, at the end of the third study block. These are designed to assist the development of analytical and application skills and the ability to present material.

Study blocks are followed by a number of placements to wards for practical consolidation of theoretical knowledge in the host authority. It was hoped initially that the different wards would be used for each of the placements to enable the sisters to observe a variety of styles of leadership and management and allow the course members to compare their own behaviour with that of their peers. Indeed, in some of the hospitals a systematic and planned ward placement is arranged at the end of each module to allow the course member to work with and observe the ward sisters of these units. However, the majority of the sisters return to their own wards between study blocks. In these instances it is hoped that the sisters will be able to look at their wards more critically and identify aspects that might require change or initiate new ideas or concepts gained from the course.

The period between the study blocks is also used in some instances to make visits and spend time with people in other parts of the hospital, for example, a day or half a day in the treasurer's department. This is particularly useful in encouraging greater understanding of other people's roles and better communication between clinical settings and support services.

A follow-up day is arranged at the end of six months for feedback and review. These sessions have included discussion of changes in members' work places which have taken place as a result of the course.

Facilitating the learning

The identification of one or more facilitators within each authority is an important feature of this scheme. The facilitators are nominated by the chief nursing officers and are managers or educationalists who act as direct links between the course members of that authority, the project director and the relevant line managers. The facilitators assist the course member to reach their course objectives and are available to give guidance and support and offer opportunities to course members in order to help the practical application of course content.

In order to establish this mechanism and orientate the facilitators to their role an early meeting was held with the nominated facilitators and project director. Subsequent meetings have taken place at regular intervals to discuss course progress and sort out any problems, as well as enabling review of the scheme. These meetings have provided opportunities for facilitators to discuss common interests and concerns with other senior nurses of the Postgraduate Teaching Hospitals and the project director.

In addition to the facilitators, the role of the project director in this scheme is very crucial as she creates the climate in which sisters can discuss and share knowledge and ideas; she acts as a leader and catalyst to the course, attempting to ensure that the group processes enhance learning and the free expression of ideas. She also helps course members to relate the more theoretical parts of the course to their particular practice setting. This link between education and service, filled by a person who is not part of the participants' hierarchy but who is seen more as an advocate, appears to be a very important aid to effective learning and performance.

OUTCOMES AND CHANGES

The general effects of the scheme are highlighted here and are discussed further in Chapter 10.

Benefits of the scheme

The scheme appears to be of benefit both to the organizations and to the individuals. In terms of the effects on the host hospitals, the planning, implementation and monitoring of the scheme has involved managers and other staff either coming together in groups to talk about the needs of sisters and how these can best be addressed, or by meeting or talking with individuals such as course members and the project director, or by providing input to the formal part of the course. Furthermore, the inclusion of all seven hospitals has fostered greater communication and cross-fertilization of information throughout the hospitals, enhanced by the discovery that similar problems exist.

One of the major ways in which such a course can provide benefits beyond those experienced by the individuals is in its capacity to increase the understanding of individuals about their role in relation to such major concerns as the provision of high-quality patient care and the power of the sister to effect change in systems for the good of patients and staff. This was often in evidence as indicated by the increased assertiveness and 'political' awareness of participants in relation to the part they play in the whole.

Despite the potential strength and power of the sister role many feel isolated (Runciman, 1983) and the opportunity to meet with their peers and discuss issues of mutual concern and interest can be of considerable benefit. This is sometimes difficult to achieve in a busy hospital setting with the day-to-day pressures of the ward work. The opportunity to spend time away from these pressures with other sisters was appreciated; for most of the participants it was the first chance they had had since their basic training to be part of a group with common experiences who were facing similar challenges.

The experience of the programme threw light on the question, For whom is such a scheme of most benefit – the staff nurse in preparation for the role of sister, the newly appointed sister who needs guidance and support in the first few months of her post, or the more experienced sister who knows what the problems are?' The flexibility and comprehensiveness of the scheme seemed to be of value to all three groups but the participants who appeared best suited were newly appointed sisters with a few months' experience in the role.

In establishing the course, attention has been paid to a wide range of nursing issues and in this respect, the course is appropriate for the different hospitals involved. It was difficult to plan the course to cater for the needs of such a mixed group. Nevertheless, although not all of the course content may be applicable in all areas of nursing, for example, theatres, outpatient departments or on night duty, the participants felt that most aspects of the course were relevant to them, notably in respect of interpersonal relationships, counselling, communications and teaching.

Participants clearly developed their knowledge and skill in many ways; for example, they gained a greater insight into the role and potential of the sister; the effective management of staff especially delegation; and an increased understanding of the issues of accountability and responsibility including the legal and ethical aspects. Moreover, a general increase in confidence was noted, as well as a shifting in attitudes of some of the sisters towards increased motivation and enthusiasm. The qualities of autonomy, creative thinking and critical appraisal are sometimes difficult to identify but there was definite evidence of changes in these attributes throughout the six months of the programme.

The weekly modular system, in contrast to a continuous block, has facilitated the release of staff whilst at the same time allowing the opportunity for the nurse to stand back from the day-to-day responsibilities of the job, unhassled by the pressures of the ward environment. The chance to reflect on the role enhances the ability to identify areas that could be developed on return to the ward or unit, and the gaps between study weeks allow time for course members to consolidate the knowledge gained during the week blocks. This pattern of training has been tried successfully with senior managers and is in line with the principle that effective learning is enhanced by the opportunity to put theory into practice and then to review the results. The modular system used in this programme allows a cycle of theory, practice and review throughout a six-month period.

Involvement in this scheme appears to have enhanced the promotion prospects of some of the participants with a number being promoted fairly soon afterwards to senior sister and senior nurse positions. Of course, it is not always clear whether this is the result of benefits gained from the course or, in the case of promotion within the hospital, the fact that the individual was made more visible by her participation in the programme and her potential thus highlighted.

Other linked developments

The experience of this scheme – focusing quite deliberately on the sister role – has paved the way for other developments including short one-week courses for senior sisters and plans for management courses, based on a similar concept, for more senior nurses. The fruitfulness of a joint training programme for a group of hospitals has been proven since there are clearly many advantages both for the individuals from the different hospitals and for the hospitals themselves.

CONCLUSION

Managers in the National Health Service are facing difficult decisions about the allocation of funds and the investment in resources. The precise relationship between programmes of this kind and factors of major importance in health care such as the improvement of standards of care, the more cost-effective provision of services, the increased motivation of staff and the decreased wastage and loss of trained manpower, are not known. However, there are indications that considerable benefits can occur from ventures such as this which have a direct bearing on many of the issues. Inevitably, if the sister, as the only nurse whose role combines a direct managerial responsibility for patients and staff, is a competent practitioner herself and one who is also able to encourage and facilitate good practice in others, this is bound to have a tremendous ripple effect.

Continuing education has suffered greatly in the past from the lack of stable funding, a fact which can in part be explained by the commonly held view that training beyond the basic qualification is at best a 'good thing' that most staff should have the opportunity to take part in at least once in their career if possible, and at worst an expensive and unnecessary luxury. If however it is viewed not just as a means of 'improving' individuals but also as a way of developing what is most valued in the organization – the best and most efficient way of providing care for patients and clients – then it should assume far greater importance in nursing than it has hitherto.

Training is not just about the provision of courses nor is the programme illustrated here necessarily the best way to meet the needs of nurses at team leader level in all health authorities. Indeed, in any case, such a programme should be only a part of a comprehensive and systematic approach to professional development which takes account of the needs of all trained staff and of the organization, and recognizes the fact that these needs are not static but dynamic. Nevertheless as long as the sister remains the key role in clinical nursing then specific investment in her continual development and support is essential.

REFERENCES

Davies, J. (1972) *A Study of Hospital Management Training in its Organisational Context: An Evaluation of First-Line Management Courses for Ward Sisters in the Manchester Region*, University of Manchester Centre of Business Research, Manchester Business School.

Davies, C. (1981) Training for ward sisters: an innovative research and development project, *Nurse Education Today*, Vol. 1, no. 2.

Dodwell, M. and Lathlean, J. (1987) An innovative training programme for ward sisters, *Journal of Advanced Nursing*, Vol. 12, pp. 311–19.

Farnish, S. (1983) *Ward Sister Preparation: A Survey in Three Districts*, NERU Report no. 2, Nursing Education Research Unit, Chelsea College, University of London.

Lathlean, J. and Farnish, S. (1984) *The Ward Sister Training Project: An Evaluation of a Training Scheme*, NERU Report no. 3, Chelsea College, University of London.

Lathlean, J., Smith, G. and Bradley, S. (1986) *Post-Registration Development Schemes Evaluation*, NERU Report no. 4, King's College, University of London.

Lelean, S. (1973) *Ready for Report, Nurse?* Royal College of Nursing, London.

Ministry of Health, Scottish Home and Health Department (1966) *Report of the Committee on Senior Nursing Staff Structure*, Chairman, B. Salmon, HMSO, London.

Redfern, S. (1981) *Hospital Sisters*, Royal College of Nursing, London.

Rogers, J. and Lawrence, J. (1987) *Continuing Professional Education for Qualified Nurses, Midwives and Health Visitors*, Ashdale Press, Peterborough.

Royal College of Nursing (1981) *A Structure for Nursing*, Royal College of Nursing, London.

Runciman, P. (1983) *Ward Sister at Work*, Churchill Livingstone, Edinburgh.

Williams, D. (1969) The administrative contribution of the nursing sister, *Public Administration*, Vol. 47. pp. 307–28.

Wood, G. (1982) Selection criteria and an outline of curriculum development, in H. Allen (ed.) *The Ward Sister: Role and Preparation*, Baillière Tindall, London.

ADDITIONAL READING

Department of Health and Social Security (1981) *The Organisation and Provision of Continuing In-Service Education and Training*, Report of the National Staff Committee for Nurses and Midwives (Chairman: B. Pattison), HMSO, London.

Dodwell, M. (1983) In-service training: 1. Continuing education in the USA; 2. On the job training in the UK, *Nursing Times*, Vol. 79, no. 24, pp. 24–6, 26–8.

Dodwell, M. (1984) A look at England and the United States, *The Journal of Continuing Education in Nursing*, Vol. 15, no. 1.

Herzberg, F. (1968) One more time: How do you motivate employees? *Harvard Business Review*, Vol. 46, p. 53.

Houle, C.O. (1961) *The Inquiring Mind*, University of Wisconsin Press, Wisconsin.

Kramer, M. and Schmalenberg, C. (1977) *Path to Biculturalism*, Nursing Resources, Wakefield, Massachusetts.

Kramer, M. (1974) *Reality Shock: Why Nurses Leave Nursing*, C.V. Mosby, St Louis.

Lysaught, J. (1972) No carrots, no sticks, *Journal of Nursing Administration*, Vol. 2, p. 43.

Maslow, A.H. (1970) *Motivation and Personality*, Harper and Row, New York.

McGregor, D. (1966) *Leadership and Motivation*, The MIT Press, Cambridge, Massachusetts.

Myers, M.S. (1964) Who are your motivated workers? *Harvard Business Review*, Vol. 42, no. 76.

Rowden, R. (1984) *Managing Nursing*, Baillière Tindall, London.

Part Two: Aspects of the Nurse's Role

3. Management of Financial Resources

Derek Reynolds

The amount spent on the National Health Service is always a contentious issue but whatever government we have it is likely that demand for services will always outstrip supply of resources. This means that choices have to be made and the resources which are available need to be managed effectively by adequately trained managers.

At every level nurses are users of resources in the NHS. In 1985/6 (according to the Health Service Costing Returns for year ended 31 March 1986) over £2.9 billion was spent on nurses' pay (i.e. 36 per cent of NHS Hospital and Community expenditure in England and Wales). Nurse managers make decisions on the deployment of nurses, the numbers required and the mix of grades and experience. They should receive some financial training to manage such a vast sum.

Nurses also make decisions which affect money spent on supplies. They may influence the choice of equipment and dressings which are used throughout a hospital. In wards and departments they use drugs, linen and other resources in their work. It is important that these decisions are made with some awareness of the financial implications. If everyone in the NHS were cost-conscious and better informed then who knows how much money would be released which could be spent, for example, on more nurses or better pay?

A further reason why nurses should be aware of financial costs is that perhaps more than any other care group they are everywhere in the organization and they see how resources are being used. For instance, they know whether their wards are overheated, whether patients are eating the food provided, and whether dressing packs contain the right items for the job. The list is endless. Managers should recognize the contribution nurses can make to financial management by involving them in discussions on value for money and by giving them budgets to manage. If nurses are to respond and to improve their contribution to management decision-making then they will benefit from financial training.

The financial training which is needed will vary according to the job being done by the nurse. This book is written for the training of nurse managers who may have had little to do with financial matters before. It is likely, therefore, that some will have only vague ideas of where the money spent in the NHS comes from and how it reaches budget-holders. Indeed, what is a budget and who decides who holds it?

This chapter tries to answer that question and contains information and guidance on sources of finance, the Körner and Griffiths recommendations and budgets.

SOURCES OF FINANCE

This section describes the sources of the money which is spent in the NHS. These sources fall within the following four headings:

- Exchequer funding
- Trust funds
- Private patient income
- Other sources.

Exchequer funding

Most of the money which is spent in the NHS comes from the taxpayer and is usually referred to as Exchequer funding. Each Autumn discussions take place between the Treasury and the DHSS about how much, in cash terms, will be allocated to health. The DHSS then decides how the cash will be distributed to Regional Health Authorities (RHAs) and a sum is set aside for the Special Health Authorities (SHAs) which do not come within the regional framework.

The cash is distributed amongst the RHAs in accordance with the RAWP formula. RAWP stands for 'Resource Allocation Working Party'. This body devised a formula in 1977 for allocating resources across the nation to achieve a fairer distribution than that which existed. The effect of this has been to move money gradually from the London region to the provinces. The formula is extremely complex and includes weightings for teaching and other relevant considerations.

It is the RHAs which decide how to allocate their funds to their District Health Authorities (DHAs).

Revenue and capital

The cash allocated by the DHSS comes in two categories, revenue and capital, and it is important to distinguish between the two because they are accounted for separately at every level in the NHS.

Revenue

Revenue cash covers recurrent expenditure such as staff pay and materials such as drugs and food.

Capital

Capital money is intended for expenditure on capital items. The definition of capital is as follows:

- Any building or engineering job costing £15,000 or more.
- Purchase of vehicles.
- Any single item of equipment costing £7,500 or more.

Some major building schemes or very expensive items of equipment are funded specifically by the DHSS/RHA/DHA as the case may be and progress is monitored by the higher authority which provided the money. These are usually referred to as 'ear-marked schemes'. Otherwise a sum of money is provided, sometimes called 'small schemes money', which managers may spend at their discretion. The policy on this varies amongst Authorities.

Trust funds

Most hospitals have trust funds. These are variously referred to as endowment monies, endowment funds or soft monies. These funds may comprise cash or investments and property bought with money donated by members of the public or from other sources. Trust funds are usually divided into general funds and specific funds or special purpose funds. The latter are often controlled by individual consultants or in some cases, nurses. Trust funds may be used for research projects or for patient or staff amenities or for the acquisition of equipment or for any other legal purpose allowed by the donor or the Authority. (In a few cases the Health Authority is not the trustee body and there are Special Trustees.) It is important that nurses or others who use these funds know that they are audited by the DHSS in exactly the same way as Exchequer monies are audited and that the Trust Fund accounts form part of the Statutory Annual Accounts of the Authority. Claims and payments must therefore be supported by adequate documentation and proper records must be maintained.

Private patient income

NHS hospitals are permitted to have a number of Private Patient (PP) beds or it may be expressed as numbers of PP days in a year. PP income is an important source of money and especially so in some hospitals which attract significant numbers of PPs. Most hospitals have not kept 'trading accounts' which show the costs of services to PPs but by-and-large the income makes a significant contribution to the cash available for NHS patients. So whatever one's views on PP medicine it is important to ensure that all PP income is collected. This is another example where nurses are ideally placed to see where there are weaknesses in the system and especially in out-patient areas where collection of income is more likely to be missed. Nurses should report their findings to managers.

Other sources of income

These are many and include public appeals; support from voluntary bodies such as the Cancer Research Campaign; income from sale of obsolete stocks or silver recovered from used X-ray film. There are many others, e.g. rents from nurses in staff residences.

Budgets

A financial budget is simply a plan expressed in financial terms. For example, the sum allocated for Community Health Services in a DHA reflects the importance which the Authority attaches to that service in its overall plan. The budget is the name given to the annual sum provided and the budget-holder is the person responsible for controlling the budget. In the past, the traditional budget-holders in a hospital have been the departmental managers (e.g. catering; domestic services); various other administrators or para-medical staff and doctors in charge of diagnostic services. High ranking nurses have held budgets for nursing costs but very few ward sisters or senior nurses have been given the responsibility of managing financial budgets. All this is changing, mostly as a result of Körner and Griffiths.

THE IMPORTANCE OF THE KÖRNER PROPOSALS

Mrs Edith Körner, a Vice-Chairman of a Regional Health Authority, was asked to head a Working Party to examine information needs in the NHS. Six reports were produced in 1982–4. They covered:

● Hospital clinical activity
● Patient transport services
● Manpower
● Miscellaneous services including radiotherapy; para-medical services; maternity services and family planning
● Community health services
● Collection and use of financial information.

The sixth report stated that it would be useful to local managers to know how much they were spending on medical specialties. This information was not available in most Authorities. While the existing financial accounts showed how much was being spent on salaries, drugs, cleaning, etc., in a District, they did not show how much was being spent on paediatrics, orthopaedics, etc. Thus 'specialty costing' was recommended. The information is far more helpful for planning purposes and is useful for generating Performance Indicators. A Performance Indicator (PI) is a measurement of performance. The commonly used 'average length of stay' is a performance indicator and is obtained by dividing the number of in-patient days by the number of in-patients. If the costs of a maternity department are divided by the number of births then the average cost of each birth can be calculated. These indicators enable managers to see, for example, that the average cost of a birth in one hospital differs from that at another hospital. The reasons can then be investigated. Similar exercises may be carried out between districts and regions.

Nursing staffing costs and the costs of what nurses do will be included in the specialty costings and they will be examined by the use of Performance Indicators. It is important, therefore, that nurses are aware of specialty costing and that they play their part in determining and justifying the costs of the specialty in which they work.

THE GRIFFITHS RECOMMENDATIONS

Sir Roy Griffiths was the man who led the team which produced the Griffiths report in 1983. The report stated that there was a lack of accountability in the NHS in that the people who used the resources, especially doctors, were not accountable for the way in which they used them. This lack of accountability extended to the management structure where no one person was in charge and accountable. The report recommended the introduction of general managers and an expansion of management budgeting. It recommended that managers who used resources should be accountable for a budget and that this included doctors – hence the term 'clinical budgeting' arose.

It follows, therefore, that where nurses use resources they should be given budgets and they should be accountable for them. The effects are to give budgets to nurses who may never have held financial budgets before. Budgets are likely to be set for wards and senior nurses and/or ward sisters may be made the budget-holders. So Griffiths has direct significance for nurses down to ward sister level as well as for nurses at top levels who have been affected personally by the appointment of general managers.

BUDGETS – WHAT DO THEY INCLUDE?

There is no set pattern for the costs which should be grouped together to form a budget. Much depends on the management structure and nurses should be encouraged to enter into local discussions. Let us take a budget for a single specialty ward for example. There will be a medical consultant at the head of the specialty. The consultant will have a 'firm' of junior doctors working under him or her and will be working with a team of nurses headed by a senior nurse and a ward sister. It is likely that the consultant's budget will include:

● Medical staff costs
● Drugs

- Charges for
  X-Ray
  Pathology
  Theatres
  Rehabilitation services.

Other costs are for discussion. Should the consultant hold the nursing budget? If he or she does it implies that the consultant controls the nursing service in that ward and is accountable for it. They may relish this but it is extremely likely that the local nursing officers would oppose it.

If budget-holders are accountable for the way their budgets are spent it is unreasonable to include items of expenditure they do not control. In our example, therefore, a single specialty ward should have two budget holders, the consultant and the nurse. The nurse should hold the budget for the nursing personnel on the ward. She should probably hold the budget for dressings and linen. Should she hold budgets for patients' meals, ward clerks, domestic staff, etc.? These considerations lead to discussions about who manages the ward clerks and the domestic staff. Should the latter answer to the ward sister or to the domestic services manager? These are all matters to be determined locally and the ward sister needs adequate financial training if she is to make a positive contribution and fight her corner if necessary.

Which nurse should be the holder of a ward budget? Should it be the senior nurse or the ward sister? Opinions on this vary and there are ward sisters who are insistent that they should hold the budgets. The general principle should be that the budget, or parts of it, should be delegated to the lowest level consistent with the responsibility held. In other words, the person who decides on the resource to be used should hold the budget for that resource.

Management Accounting Department

It is usually the job of the Management Accounts section of the Finance Department to liaise with budget-holders. It should be there to help budget-holders and nurses who are given budgets should work at establishing a close relationship with the Management Accounting staff as this will be useful to both sides. Management Accounts will benefit from being kept in touch with what is happening at the front line and throughout the organization. This is not only useful to their work but it should provide them with enhanced job satisfaction as they can relate what they are doing to what is happening with patients. In return the nurse will receive guidance and support and should make more effective use of the resources available. This is not only achieved by the management accountant telling the nurse each month how much she has spent but also by costing alternative solutions to problems which nurses may be considering.

Budget-setting

Budgets should be set by the management accountant and the nurse sitting down together and discussing the nurse's work plan for the ensuing financial year. When this conversation takes place will vary from Authority to Authority and it will be timed to fit in with the planning procedure and timetable used by the Authority. When the management accountant has costed the proposals agreed with the nurse they will be added to all the other bids from budget-holders. It is likely that the aggregated bids will exceed the money available and there will be considerable negotiation going on at various levels until decisions are made on the final budgets to be allocated. Nurse budget-holders must be capable of arguing their cases and supporting them with factual information including costs. They must also be prepared to say and to justify to managers at the outset that for a certain cost a certain level of service can be provided. It is then for the manager to decide on the priorities and on the level of service which is required.

Budget reports

Budget reports usually take the form of monthly statements prepared by Management Accounts and given to budget-holders as soon after the end of the month to which they relate. The sooner this is the better chance there is of taking effective remedial action, if such action is called for. Budget-holders should not wait longer than three weeks for their statements and they should press to have the time shortened to that which is reasonably possible.

An example of a typical and simple statement is given in Table 3.1.

Table 3.1   An example of a monthly statement

Histopathology		1986/7 October (month 7)[1]		
Expenditure head[2]	Annual budget[3]	Budget for period[4]	Expenditure for period[5]	Over/ under[6]
Staff	70,000	41,000	38,500	2,500
Supplies				
Lab. materials	7,000	4,000	5,900	(1,900)
Lab. equipment	2,000	1,200	500	700
Med. & tech. journals	700	400	300	100
	79,700	46,600	45,200	1,400

[1] In the NHS, finance staff invariably refer to the months in the financial year by numbers, thus, April is month 1, May is month 2 and so on. October is month 7.
[2] The expenditure head is the description of the type of expenditure incurred. There is an increasing tendency towards computerized accounting systems which allow these to be tailor-made to the individual requirements of budget-holders.
[3] The annual budget is the sum allocated for the entire year.
[4] 'Budget for the period' is the sum allocated for the period 1 April to the end of the report, i.e. October in this example. It is usual to phase the annual budget for staff pay in equal monthly amounts throughout the year because it reflects the manner in which the expenditure is incurred. This pattern may not be true for supplies items. Gas and electricity bills for example may be paid quarterly and the budget should reflect this, otherwise there will be an underspend or an overspend shown almost every month.
[5] This relates to the same period as 4 above. Budget-holders should check what this figure actually covers. Is it simply the *cash* which has been paid out or does it include items which have been *ordered and not yet paid for*, i.e. *commitments*? If it does not include commitments then it is not as helpful as it might be and budget-holders should be aware of it because it does not reflect the true position.
[6] This is the 'variance' being the difference between the budget for the period and the expenditure for the period.

Variances

There are many reasons for variances, e.g.

● The budget was incorrectly set in the first place.
● The phasing of the expenditure over the year is wrong.
● The activity was more/less than expected.
● Pay awards or price increases have not been provided for.

The important point is that budget-holders should be aware of the variances and the reasons for them.

What happens if I overspend?

The answer to this question depends upon the cause of the overspend. If a ward budget is overspent it may be caused by higher than expected activity. In this case it is for management to decide whether to accept this level of activity, in which case the budget should be increased or permitted to overspend. If activity is not the answer then the overspend may be caused by price increases of goods and materials or changes in working practices. In these cases the budget-holder must review what is being used or how things are done and whether changes can be made to stay within budget or whether a case may be made for seeking an increase. The management accountant may be helpful in these circumstances.

What happens if I underspend?

Once again the answer depends on the cause. It is quite possible to stay within the cash sum allocated to a budget-holder and still achieve poor value for money if the activity levels fall. The budget-holder should always look at activity as well as the cash spent.

It could be that posts have not been filled because staff could not be recruited.

In either of these cases it is likely that the Finance Department will want to claw-back all or some of the underspend and redeploy the money elsewhere. The budget-holder should not feel threatened by this necessarily, provided it is understood and agreed that a temporary underspend is indeed temporary and that the funding will be restored when the position has changed.

If, however, budget-holders take positive management action to save money, then they must be allowed to keep it in their department or at least receive preferential consideration when management decides how to use it. Thus, if the budget-holder is a ward sister who proposes to hold a vacancy for a month in order to save enough money for a bed hoist, then she should discuss it in advance with Management Accounts so that the position is understood at the outset. Such incentives must be part of the budgetary system if budget-holders are to be encouraged to seek improved value for money.

In short if the underspend is *planned* the budget-holder has an entitlement to it. If it is fortuitous or outside the budget-holders' control then they have no inalienable right to keep it.

Virement

Moving money from one part of a budget to another is called 'virement'. Budget-holders should ascertain the local rules on the power of virement as some Authorities allow budget-holders to vire sums up to a certain level within their budgets.

SUMMARY

Nurses are not angels of mercy but professional people who are in an ideal position to make an important contribution to the management process at all levels of the NHS. General managers who are not nurses do well to involve nurses in management and in decision-making. If nurses are to respond to the challenge then their professional skills need to be developed to encompass a greater understanding of resource management.

This chapter has provided guidance on sources of finance and on control of budgets but above all it has attempted to encourage communication between the nursing and accountancy professions. Between them they can make a massive contribution to the more effective use of limited resources which will help staff and patients alike.

REFERENCES AND USEFUL READING

Department of Health and Social Security (1976) *Sharing Resources for Health in England: Report of the Resource Allocation Working Party*, HMSO, London.

Department of Health and Social Security (1982) *Report of the NHS/DHSS Steering Group on Health Services Information* (Körner Report), HMSO, London.

Department of Health and Social Security (1983) *NHS Management Inquiry Report* (Griffiths Report), HMSO, London.

Jones, T. and Prowle, M. (1987) *Health Service Finance: An Introduction* (3rd edn), The Certified Accountants Educational Trust, London.

The National Association of Health Authorities (NAHA) (1987) *NHS Handbook* (3rd edn), The Macmillan Press Ltd, London, particularly Section 2: Finance and information.

4. The Planning Process and Manpower Resources

Jane Burrows

THE PLANNING PROCESS WITHIN THE NHS

Introduction

When considering the range and complexity of services which an average District Health Authority has to run within a cash limited budget, it is essential that the spending of that budget is planned in a systematic way in order to achieve service objectives and spend that money in the most effective way. In order to facilitate the optimal use of available resources the NHS introduced a formalized planning system in 1976[1] which required regions and districts to produce long- and short-term comprehensive plans.

What is planning?

Any planning process is concerned with four questions:

- Where are we now?
- Where do we want to be?
- How do we get there?
- How are we doing?

Where are we now?
This requires the need for a district profile to be written, which contains

basic information about the health district:

- Description of the population served,
- Current service provision and policy,
- Current manpower resource and distribution,
- Current estate,
- Current expenditure pattern.

Description of the population served

This information will include data on the following: a definition and measurement of the catchment population, the age/sex structure of that population, social-class distribution, presence of ethnic minorities, areas of deprivation, poor housing, number of homeless, single-parent families, mortality rates in the form of Standard Mortality Ratio (SMR) main causes of death and an idea of morbidity rates and the perinatal mortality rate.

Current service provision and policy

This section of the profile would contain details of the current service provision provided by care group, i.e. acute, elderly, mental illness, etc. in terms of number of beds/places, cases treated, throughput, occupancy levels, etc. with a description of overall clinical policy by care group.

Current manpower resource and distribution

This should contain the current number of staff by discipline, grade, sex, age distribution, full-time/part-time, by care group where possible. Obviously nursing and medical staff are easier to attach to a specific care group than works or ancillary staff, who are likely to be attached to hospital sites rather than specific care groups.

Current estate

This would contain a detailed measurement of the capital estate, which includes the numbers and type of buildings in the district, space availability, value, the condition in terms of maintenance and repair and an assessment of the functional suitability of the building for its current and potential usage.

Current expenditure pattern

This would be a cost statement of the current pattern of expenditure in revenue and capital terms. Revenue is the expenditure on actually running services and is therefore recurring every year, whereas capital is the allocation spent on buildings either in new build, renovation, repair and re-use of existing buildings, and is a one-off expenditure and, therefore, non-recurring.

This assessment of the current situation can be one of the most difficult aspects of the planning process, as there is an enormous amount of data to collect in a form appropriate for planning. It can take officers several months to collect but once completed can be reasonably straight-forward to update.

Where do we want to be?

This is the area of planning where close scrutiny of the data on the population to be served is essential and planning decisions should relate closely to population need. For example if the age structure shows a higher than average elderly population, then a higher volume of service to the elderly in terms of community support, day care and beds would be required. An inner-city district with areas of deprivation may well require a larger volume and range of community services than a district within a relatively affluent area.

It is at this stage of strategic planning where the volume and quality of care to be provided at year 10 has to be agreed and tailored to expected financial resources. Decisions on care policies should be agreed and the location and manpower requirements and potential costs of the services defined. Working within potential financial constraints may require the rationalization of some services to allow for development of other services.

How do we get there?

Once the picture of the service in ten years' time is decided and agreed, the steps towards achieving these objectives then have to be planned in the most appropriate time-scale. There may well be constraints in terms of time scale such as the actual financial allocation or the need to provide a new capital development.

The planned steps towards the strategic objective are necessarily less clearly defined from years 5–10 but years 1–2 will be described in detail and be achievable within the financial allocation. Years 3–5 will be reasonably firm but may include contingency plans for a plus or a minus 2 per cent option if the financial allocation is not realized.

How are we doing?

This is the stage of the planning process which monitors and measures the achievement of the objectives set out in the annual/short-term plan

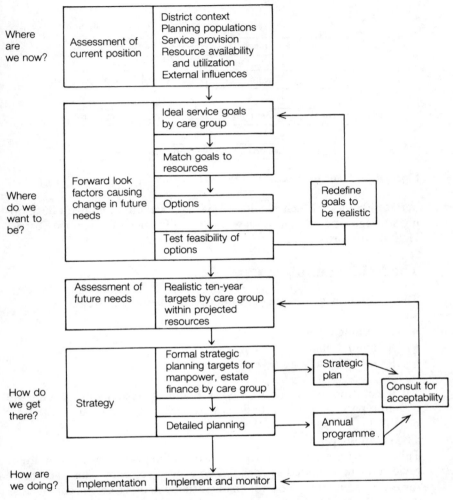

Source: Centre for Health Services Management, Leicester Polytechnic

Figure 4.1 Planning process – Mereworth approach

against the broader objectives of the strategic/long-term plan on an annual basis.

This planning process is well illustrated by the Mereworth approach (Figure 4.1), which was developed by the Centre for Health Service Management, Leicester Polytechnic, as a training model for Health

PROCESS

NHS system

```
┌─────────────────────────┐
│    Where are we now?     │───────────┐
└─────────────────────────┘           │
            ↓                          │
┌─────────────────────────┐    ┌──────────────────┐
│   Where do we want to be │──▷ │  Strategic plan  │
└─────────────────────────┘    └──────────────────┘
            ↓                          │
┌─────────────────────────┐    ┌──────────────┐
│    How do we get there   │───────────────▷│  Annual plan │
└─────────────────────────┘    └──────────────┘
            ↓
┌─────────────────────────┐    ┌─────────────────────────┐
│    How are we doing?     │──▷ │  Annual planning review │
└─────────────────────────┘    └─────────────────────────┘
```

Figure 4.2 Planning process and the NHS system

Service Planners, which provided a systematic methodology for developing strategic and annual plans within fixed financial limits for a District Health Authority.

The NHS planning system

There are 3 distinct elements to the NHS Planning System:

● The strategic plan,
● The annual plan,
● The annual planning review process.

An illustration as to how the NHS Planning System fits in with the planning process, previously described, is shown in Figure 4.2.

The strategic plan
This is a long-term plan covering a period of ten years, which is rewritten, reviewed and amended as appropriate every five years. This five-yearly review is essential to allow for changes that will inevitably occur, such as new medical technology, the economic climate which will affect expected resource allocation and manpower availability.

The strategic plan is a comprehensive plan for all services provided at district level, which identifies and describes service goals and objectives for each care group, and identifies manpower and any capital development required to achieve those objectives.

Finally plans are fully costed and have to be tailored to match an overall expected financial allocation, and because of the difficulty in forecasting future finance ten years ahead, can be approached on a contingency basis such as on existing levels, plus and minus 2 per cent of current financial allocation.

It is important that the strategic plan is realistic and all potential constraints identified.

All districts produce a strategic plan which then form the basis for the regional strategic plan. It should be noted that Special Health Authorities (SHAs) do not come within the regional network and plans are sent directly to the DHSS.

Prior to districts writing their strategic plan, guidelines are distributed by region to districts in order to identify broad parameters within which to plan; these would include national and regional priorities such as development of community services for mental illness and mental handicap services and the contraction of large institutions. Service targets, such as number of beds and expected caseloads by care group, would be identified. The strategic plan is, therefore, a comprehensive plan, describing in broad overall terms where the service within that district expects to be in ten years' time. It states 'Where are we now?' by an assessment of the current situation and the plan fully describes 'Where do we want to be?' by care group and 'How do we get there?' in broad terms.

The annual plan

This plan is written annually and covers year 1 in detail against firm manpower, capital and financial resources. Year 2 is described against expected resources, in detail but less firm than year 1. Any expected changes in services whether expanding or contracting are matched with manpower, capital and financial implications, which incorporate any development monies and cost improvements (savings). The annual plan sets out the detailed objectives for the district by care group and therefore describes the planning stage of 'How do we get there?' The annual plan is monitored at the end of the year and it is possible then to identify whether the objectives have been achieved or not.

On receipt of all the district annual plans, the region then analyses all the district plans in order to produce a regional annual plan which is forwarded to the DHSS for analysis and monitoring through the review process.

The annual planning review process

This is the monitoring procedure by which the annual plan proposals are measured against what has actually happened at the end of planning year 1.

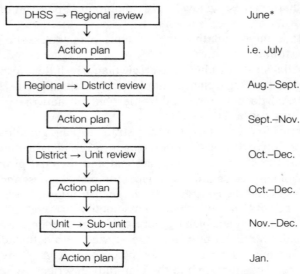

DHSS → Regional review	June*
↓	
Action plan	i.e. July
↓	
Regional → District review	Aug.–Sept.
↓	
Action plan	Sept.–Nov.
↓	
District → Unit review	Oct.–Dec.
↓	
Action plan	Oct.–Dec.
↓	
Unit → Sub-unit	Nov.–Dec.
↓	
Action plan	Jan.

* The Timetable example depends on the timing of the DHSS → Regional Review.

Figure 4.3   Annual planning review process

This procedure, held annually, commences with the DHSS reviewing the regional performance against the objectives and targets set in the regional annual plan. This results in an agreed action plan which is then measured against achievements in the following year. This review process describes the monitoring stage of 'How are we doing?'

The region then repeats the process (within approximately three months) with all districts, again producing an agreed action plan. The districts then repeat the process with the units and increasingly the units are now repeating the process with the sub units (see Figure 4.3). This process indicates a 'top down' monitoring procedure whereas the actual planning process is a 'bottom up' procedure in that the units and districts compile a plan both strategic and annual, which is then aggregated into regional and then national plans.

Performance indicators

The development of Performance Indicators (PIs) was introduced by the DHSS in 1983/4.[2] This was an attempt to introduce measures or indicators of performance comparison by care group between regions and between districts. These indicators are still in early stages of development

Total DHA nursing & midwifery staff
M8   % Non-med. staff WTE – N&M
M14   % Total staff cost – N&M
MM21   Average cost/WTE – N&M
MM27   Staff WTE/IP case – N&M

Nursing staff – acute services
M39A   % Total nurses (acute) – trained
M39B   % Total nurses (acute) – learner
M39C   % Total nurses (acute) – auxil.
M40   Total nurses (acute)/occ. bed
M41   Total nurses (acute)/avail. bed

Nursing staff – mental illness
M45A   % Total nurses (MI) – trained
M45B   % Total nurses (MI) – learner
M45C   % Total nurses (MI) – auxil.
M46   Total nurses (MI)/occ. bed
M47   Total nurses (MI)/avail. bed

Nursing & midwifery staff – maternity
M56A   % Maternity nursing staff – midwives
M56B   % Maternity nursing staff – trained
M56C   % Maternity nursing staff – learner
M56D   % Maternity nursing staff – auxil.
M57   Maternity WTE/100 DHA births

Nursing staff – child care
C1   Reg. nurses in SCBUs/100 births
C2   Reg. nurses in SCBUs/SCBU case
C43   Health Visitor contact rate – 1–4 yrs
C44   Health Visitors/1000 under-5s
C45   Health Visiting staff/1000 under-5s
C55   Nurse/occupied paediatric bed – SRNs
C56   Nurse/occupied paediatric bed – other

Nursing staff – community services
M53A   % Community nursing staff – DN & HV
M53B   % Community nursing staff – trained
M53C   % Community nursing staff – auxil.
M54   Total community nursing/1000 pop.
M15   CPN & day hospital nursing/100,000 pop.
MH16   CMHNs/100,000 resident pop.

Health-visiting staff – by DHA
M52A   % Health-visiting staff – Health Visitors
M52B   %Health-visiting staff – trained
M52C   % Health-visiting staff – auxil.
C43   Health-visitor contact rate – 1–4 yrs
C44   Health Visitors/1000 under-5s
C45   Health-visiting staff/1000 under-5s
E6   Health-visiting contact rate – 65+ yrs

Source: *Performance Indicators for the NHS,* DHSS, London, published annually since
1982/3.

and are utilized to identify and compare a district's performance against other districts, both regionally and nationally and to 'flag up' 'outliers', such as those lying 10 per cent above or below the national average. They do not provide answers but raise questions in order to challenge. An example of some of the nursing indicators are as shown in Table 4.1.

Capital planning

A strategic plan will often highlight capital deficiencies due to policy changes or inappropriate existing buildings. For example, due to a policy to contract the large mental illness institutions and develop comprehensive district services, a need for an acute mental illness unit may be a requirement in the district in order to achieve a comprehensive range of services in the district by year 10. This objective will initiate an option appraisal[3] which is the first stage of the capital planning process as described in Capricode[4] which is a guide issued by the DHSS, detailing a systematic procedure for the planning, building, commissioning and evaluation of a capital project.

Option appraisal

This is a systematic attempt to specify and compare options or alternatives for meeting stated objectives. It involves making more explicit the commonsense process of taking into account all the major costs and benefits of alternative solutions to a problem before committing resources to a project.

Stages of option appraisal analysis

- Definition of objectives – i.e. to attain comprehensive services for the mentally ill within the district.
- Alternatives for achieving those objectives:
  Increased community support,
  Staffed residential provision in the community,
  Day care, joint financing with Local Authority,
  Upgrade existing building,
  New DGH unit compatible with resource assumptions.
- Draw up a shortlist of options with: costs, manpower and other revenue implications, capital implications, and the benefits and disadvantages of each option.

Stages of capital planning

- Briefing,
- Design,
- Production drawings,
- Construction,
- Commissioning,
- Evaluation.

Once a decision has been taken to build a new unit, a project team is set up. This can be divided into two distinct groups, which must work closely together:

- Client group consisting of doctors, nurses, health planners, suppliers, and personnel.
- Technical group consisting of architects, engineers, quantity surveyors.

The function of the client group is to provide a brief and the function of the technical group is to interpret the brief in building terms.

A brief is defined as issuing instructions to the design team stating requirements which have to be met by the buildings being planned. Those requirements will be defined firstly by operational policies which form the basis of the brief. A policy is defined as an agreed method of operation of service or department in terms of its functional requirement and the implications for design and staffing.

There are 3 types of policy:

- Whole hospital – this is an explanation of how different departments relate and how whole hospital services such as catering, portering, engineering, security, etc. will function.
- Operational – department/ward – this is an explanation of how the department/ward is expected to work, the type of patient, nursing and medical requirements, etc.
- An operational manual is a detailed district commissioning document which fills in the specific detail and requirements of how the wards and departments are expected to function at the commissioning stage. It also gives advice on the furnishing and equipment of wards and departments.

Implications for the ward/department sister and the nurse team leader in the community

The strategic plan

Nurses at operational level should always make a point of reading their district's strategic plan, in order to be aware of the particular needs and of the population served by the district, the overall direction and objectives set for the next ten years, and the implications for the nurses' specific unit within that plan. This will enable the nurse to participate in the planning process and suggest ideas for implementing that strategy. The nurse should always be aware of the timing of the five-year review of the strategic plan, so that he/she can contribute to the unit input, particularly in relation to potential changes in clinical practice and nursing care.

The annual plan

Nurses are able to contribute to the detail required within the annual plan, for example to define manpower implications in order to achieve an extra caseload target. The nurse is ideally suited to identifying manpower implications for both development and rationalization/contracting situations.

The annual review

The nurse at operational level should be involved in the unit→sub-unit review and should be capable of monitoring his/her ward/department against an agreed action plan from the previous year. The nurse will also become increasingly involved in quality assurance and help to develop indicators to measure quality. The nurse should also be aware of how the district and unit stand in the Performance Indicator package against the national scene, and should annually request a printout of the PI package following its distribution to all districts in January.

Capital planning

The nurse is a crucial contributor to the briefing team, particularly in the writing of the operational policies. The nurse should also be able to make comments on initial sketch plans, space requirements and critical dimensions, such as those required for elderly patients and advise on practical room and departmental relationships, such as X-ray sited next to the Accident and Emergency Department or the relationship of clean utility to the treatment room.

PLANNING AND MANAGING THE MANPOWER RESOURCE

Manpower accounts for approximately 75 per cent of the total NHS revenue expenditure and nurse manpower represents approximately 47 per cent of that total staffing expenditure and around 70 per cent of the total NHS workforce. Therefore nurse manpower is a critical factor to consider when it comes to assessing the implications of planning services around an estimated need and monitoring manpower expenditure.

The importance of good manpower planning and control was emphasized by the National Audit Office[5] and the Committee of Public Accounts[6] and both reports were critical of the lack of planning and control of nurse manpower within the NHS.

Manpower planning – what is it?

Manpower planning like any other planning process is concerned with the four questions described on p. 52 of this chapter.

Where are we now?

This question provokes the need for a sound and accurate data base and is an area where the NHS, until recently, has failed to realize the importance of an up-to-date and accurate data base for identifying current numbers of staff. The data should be divided into disciplines by care group, sex, full-time, part-time, grade, etc. Age structures, wastage rates, sickness rates, length of time in post, qualifications, etc. are other items of information which the nurse manager at ward/department, unit level and above require for adequate monitoring.

Many districts are in the process of developing or have developed a comprehensive system for providing managers with details of current staff-in-post as described above. The DHSS collect information twice a year called census data, which they utilize to monitor nurse staffing and it also forms the basis for the Performance Indicator manpower information.

Once the manpower data base is established it is then possible to draw a simple manpower system chart, which illustrates current staff in post by grade, and the in and out flows of that manpower system in terms of starters, qualified, unqualified and learners. The outflow should, of course, include retirements, transfers and promotions. The manpower system chart should be drawn to scale so that the boxes and the widths of

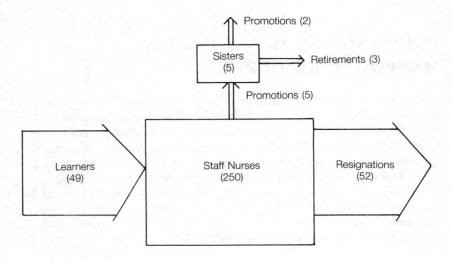

Figure 4.4 A manpower system

flow are directly in visual proportion to each other.

See Figure 4.4 (A manpower system), which illustrates a simple system of identifying qualifying learners, staff nurse and sisters. It is clear from Figure 4.4 that the problem is one of replacing the wastage that occurs at staff nurse level and not of finding candidates suitable for promotion. One option would be to recruit staff nurses from other districts other than from the qualifying learners. There are three basic factors common to all manpower systems:

● the level of demand,
● the rate of loss,
● the replacement policy.

The assessment of these three factors has become a major part of an effective approach to managing the manpower resource.[7]

The essential factors of a manpower supply model, therefore, are numbers of staff in post by grade, numbers recruited (annually), wastage numbers (annually), number of promotions and an age distribution of staff. All numbers should be expressed in whole time equivalents (wte).

Where do we want to be?
One of the most fundamental elements in nurse manpower planning is the assessment of nursing demand. This has always been a controversial issue

as to what is the best and most acceptable method. The Public Accounts Committee[8] stressed the importance of utilizing a demand estimation method. Historically the NHS has had a 'best guess' at estimating the numbers of nurses required and has heavily relied on the sister's judgement without utilizing a systematic approach. There are two types of Demand Methodology:

Top-down method
This method is utilized for strategic planning purposes and is a broad estimate of nurse manpower requirements usually in the form of a 'norm', i.e. one nurse for 1.18 beds. Top-down approaches are normally only applied from 'above', i.e. regions analysing hospital data. The statistical basis for the formulae requires a large data base in order to obtain significant results. A regression formula is often used to provide 'expected' staffing levels from levels of activity to show workload achieved and also identifies unexplained differences in staffing between hospitals or districts. Problems of acceptability of a 'top-down' approach, are that the standard or norm suggested by national or regional current average staffing levels may be considered inappropriate to individual districts or hospitals.

The measurement of workload may be considered incorrect, for instance where the number of available beds in a district or hospital have very high occupancy levels. It is also questionable whether a 'top-down' approach can take account of all aspects of workload.

Other disadvantages of a norm-based method are that they tend not to contain any explicit scientific assessment of workload or standard of care.

The advantages of top-down and norm-based methods are that they are quick and easy to apply and are useful for estimating staffing requirements for new developments.

Bottom-up method
These are for the purpose of day-to-day allocation of nursing staff to meet requirements on a short-term basis. These methods all collect data from a ward base. There are two main types of bottom-up methods:

- Dependency methods, such as Cheltenham, Leicester, Oxford and the Northern Dependency methods;
- Consultative methods, such as Telford or the Brighton modification of Telford.

All these methods have been fully described and evaluated by the DHSS Operational Research Service.[9]

Dependency methods are characterized by developing means of classifying patients which relate to how much nursing care they need, i.e. the dependency of a patient.

The disadvantages are:

- They tend to produce ideal staffing levels irrespective of financial constraints.
- They are also time-consuming and costly to implement.
- There is little account, for instance of counselling and psychiatric elements of care and broad assumptions are made regarding standardization of procedures.

Consultative methods, such as the Brighton and Telford systems, rely basically on the professional judgement of the ward sister and her team to identify safe and acceptable levels of staffing, which in discussion are then challenged by the local nurse managers. The advantages of this system are that it is relatively simple, flexible and cheap to implement.

The disadvantage is it is based on subjective assessment.

It should be noted, however, that all methodologies rely on an element of professional judgement, which implies that subjectivity forms part of all assessment of patient care. Once the numbers of nurses required are identified, thought should then be given to the issue of skill mix[10] and at least the ratio of trained to untrained staff should be identified for each care group.

The plan should then be costed to ascertain whether it comes within the expected financial parameters.

Training implications should also be identified in outline at this stage. For example if it is expected that more RMNs and CPNs will be required at the end of the planning period, extra intakes or placements will need to be identified at the appropriate time. The manpower plan may also identify a need for redeployment, for instance nurses may need to move from the large mental illness and handicap-contracting institutions into the community and this will also produce a requirement for reorientation training for staff.

How do we get there?

Once the current manpower situation and the expected demand are quantified, it is then possible to identify the gap between 'Where are we now?' as against 'Where do we want to be?' It is identifying the means of closing this gap between demand and supply that will determine 'How do we get there?' The manpower changes, which might be a mixture of increase, decrease and redeployment of staff, should be measured on an annual basis, so that at the end of the planning period the target figures should be achieved.

These annual steps should be thought/through in detail and should be realistic in financial and operational terms. The future supply of nurses should also be assessed at this stage and tested to see whether it will match the demand. The training implications noted above should be programmed in at the appropriate planning year.

How are we doing?

This is the monitoring stage of the process, in which we measure what actually happened in year 1 against the planned out-turn for year 1. If the objectives were not achieved, thought has to be given as to how the situation can be redressed in future years and the annual plans amended accordingly.

The Performance Indicator manpower package is also useful to examine in conjunction with monitoring the annual manpower plan, as it is possible to compare one district against other districts, one region against others, also regionally and nationally – an example of some of the Nurse Manpower Performance Indicators is shown in Figure 4.4.

Managing the manpower resource at ward/department/ community level

The key figure determining the quality and cost-effectiveness of care is the leader of the ward nursing team,[11] the sister/charge nurse in charge of a department such as OPD and the sister-in-charge of the community nursing teams. One of the factors of crucial importance is that the ward/department leader has relevant, appropriate and up-to-date management and financial information in order to manage the ward/ department/community team in the most cost-effective way.

Information required

Budget statements

These should be obtainable from the unit treasurer and the sister should discuss the format and the information required in that statement with the Treasurer. The information should contain the establishment in whole time equivalents (wte) by Grade with the costs of salaries paid including overtime payments. The funded establishment should also be stated, which is the agreed establishment with minus a 1 per cent or 2 per cent vacancy factor included depending on local policy. Some establishments may be fully funded without a vacancy factor being deducted.

The sister should be aware of the total annual manpower budget for the ward/department and should have participated with management in the setting up of the ward establishment and the grade mix.

Monthly expenditure statements

These should also be provided by the unit treasurer to enable the sister/charge nurse to monitor the staffing expenditure monthly against the annual budget.

Overspending may be caused by:

- over exceeding the funded establishment;
- change in the grade mix, i.e. increase in qualified staff;
- incremental payments – this is when a number of staff are on the maximum increment;
- overtime payments;
- too many qualified staff at weekends when the workload is lower;
- high use of agency staff.

It is important that the sister can identify the causes of overspending and underspending on her ward/department.

Wastage and sickness rates

The sister should keep records of staff who leave and abnormal sickness rates. Many districts now have computerized systems for collating personnel information, which will provide regular statements of staff movement, but if not the nurse managers and ward sisters should collate the information manually. A high rate of wastage or sickness may be an indication of low morale on the ward, which would require investigation as to the cause.

Workload measurements

It is very advantageous to collect regular information on dependency levels in order to reflect workload implications, which can then be utilized to plan a better match between manpower availability and the workload. If it is obvious that the workload is going to be too high for the number of nurses available in a certain week, this information on workload measurement and staff availability can be discussed with clinicians, so that it may be possible to alter the workload by amending planned admissions or altering a theatre session to help alleviate a potential crisis.

Duty rotas

These should be drawn carefully to plan for as good a match of staff against projected workload as possible. Staff should be utilized flexibly and some of the most successful reductions of overlaps have occurred when it has been left to the sister to work out with her staff the best way to provide an even deployment of nurses, rather than having a district-wide imposed shift system. Some nurses find it convenient to work a split shift. Others appreciate a flexi-time system, which can assist efforts to attain a more even distribution of staff throughout the week. The correct level and grade of staff should be planned at weekends, when often the number and dependency of patients tend to be lower and therefore require less qualified staff.

There is a move towards designating an increasing number of wards as five-day and day-care wards. These considerably reduce staff expenditure.

Management budgeting

One of the recommendations of the Griffiths report was concerned with the development and setting of management budgets and the involvement of clinicians in management as it is they who control the amount of resources needed and used in treatment and care.

Management budgeting is about management rather than accounts. The major objectives being to provide a better service to NHS clients by helping clinicians and nurse managers to make better informed judgements about how the resources they control can be used to the maximum effect. A responsibility accounting approach is used so that costs and recharges are passed from one manager to another. There are three types of manager.

- *User budget-holders* – clinicians who are charged for the services and resources they use for patients.
- *Facility budget-holders* – sisters/charge nurses who manage wards and departments, will charge clinicians as user budget-holders for nursing time, treatments, bed use, etc. Facility budgets will also show charges to that budget from other departments such as catering, pharmacy and CSSD.

● *Departmental budget-holders* i.e. CSSD, catering, radiology, physiotherapy, etc. will charge wards and departments for their products and services.[12]

Various pilot projects have been set up throughout the country in order to test the concept and to develop a functional set of management information from which consultants, ward sisters and others can manage their wards and departments in the most cost-effective way.

This chapter has not attempted to discuss the important issues of quality of care, and leadership style, both of which are crucial factors in the management of the ward or department. Quality is an area of which all staff should be concerned and should all participate as a team in setting standards of care. Finally, the current pressures for high performance levels, combined with high quality of care, means that ward sisters must motivate their staff and gain their commitment and participation towards attaining high standards.

NOTES

1. NHS Planning System Circular HC(76)29.
2. Performance Indicators HN(83)25.
3. Option Appraisal HN(81)30.
4. Capricode HN(86)32.
5. NAO (National Audit Office), NHS, *Control of Nursing Manpower*, HMSO, London, 1985.
6. PAC, *Committee of Public Accounts 14th Report*, HMSO, London, 1985.
7. Malcolm Bennison and Jonathan Cosson, Institute of Manpower Studies, *The Manpower Planning Handbook*, McGraw-Hill, Maidenhead, 1984.
8. See note 6.
9. ORS Critique, *A Critique of Methods for Determining Nurse Staffing Levels in Hospitals*, DHSS, London, 1985.
10. *Mix and Match of Review of Nursing Skill Mix,* DHSS, London, February 1986.
11. *Managing the Manpower Future Part 1,* DHSS, London, 1981.
12. Angela Abbott, Developing a management budget, *Nursing Times*, Vol. 82, no. 4, pp. 46–7.

5. Staff Appraisal and Performance Review

Tom Kerrane

INTRODUCTION

Simple, yet meaningful, definitions of 'management' are limited and therefore the following retain their value:

- 'Getting things done through people' or
- 'Deciding what needs to be done and then getting someone else to do it'.

All managers are involved with setting aims or objectives for their organization and then making the best possible use of all their resources in order to achieve these agreed aims. The manager is often described as an 'enabler' with a key task of developing the knowledge and skills of all the people who work for him.

To carry this out effectively requires a mechanism whereby each member of the organization is appraised by their immediate manager on a regular basis. Strengths and weaknesses are identified and personal objectives are agreed. We are now describing the 'appraisal' system which is recognized as a major tool of sound management in any field or organization. The individual has a basic need to be told 'how he or she is getting on' in their work.

The introduction of a sound appraisal and performance review system can represent a most positive strategy for meeting goals and assisting the individual to develop. Within the National Health Service, both in the hospital and community settings, a good appraisal scheme can bring enormous benefits to nurses at all levels and to standards of patient care.

Appraisal therefore can be described simply as a component of good management practice. We are meeting the needs of the individual who is asking:

- Tell me what you expect of me.
- Tell me how I am doing.
- Guide me and help me to improve my performance.
- Give me an opportunity to perform better.

The appraisal system, centred around a well-structured interview, can focus on each of these needs and ensure that there is a positive development plan for each worker within the organization. The appraisal interview provides the manager with a valuable opportunity to talk openly to a member of staff. They can learn of problems within their department which are causing frustration to staff, in addition to learning of factors which will increase motivation. For the appraisee, the interview is also an opportunity to hear first-hand how he or she is perceived by the manager. Have their additional efforts been recognized? Will there be any reward for success? How can he be helped to improve over the next year?

THE INDUSTRIAL SCENE

Appraisal systems have been in use within industrial settings for many years as a means of monitoring and reviewing the performance of workers at all levels. These systems, in various degrees of sophistication, are normally linked directly with salary increases. Attempts are made to assess workers against a number of defined qualities. For example:

- Knowledge of the job
- Accuracy
- Productivity
- Overall job performance
- Industriousness
- Initiative
- Judgement
- Co-operation
- Personality
- Versatility

In recent years, some doubts have been expressed about the means used to assess some of these qualities and a number of organizations are experimenting with new approaches to appraisal systems. It is recognized that it is important to distinguish merit-rating plans, which may stress the personal qualities and contribution of the individual, from job evaluation plans which are concerned with assessments of job content and job requirements rather than the person doing it. Experience has shown that the actual objective measurement of working performance is often extremely difficult.

Peter Drucker, the American management consultant and prolific author of many books on management, is convinced that every organization requires an appraisal system. He is critical, however, of those who use an empty mechanistic approach to the appraisal procedure and fail to use it as an integral component of effective man-management. Drucker describes the executives who complete the yearly appraisal form on each of their subordinates and then proceed to file it away as just another piece of useless paper. One clue to what is wrong was contained in an advertisement of a new book on management in America which talked of the appraisal interview as 'a most distasteful job' for the manager.

He believes that the effective appraisal should focus on a number of key questions:

- What has he done well?
- What, therefore, is he likely to be able to do well?
- What does he have to learn or to acquire to be able to get the full benefit from his strength?
- 'If I had a son or daughter, would I be willing to have him or her work under this person?'
  If yes, why?
  If no, why?

This approach makes one look closely at the *individual*. Personal strengths are clearly identified and weaknesses can be seen as limitations to the maximum use of his strengths and future potential.

It is understandable that there has been a tendency in some organizations for job performance evaluations to become one-sided procedures by which a supervisor measures an employee against pre-established criteria. Although this remains valuable for management, it could lead to a situation whereby the worker becomes totally passive and regards the appraisal mechanism as one-sided and not requiring his active participation. In both industrial and other settings, systems must be constantly under review to ensure that they offer a framework for individuals to be both assessed and developed in parallel.

Each of us benefits by taking time to explore what, how and why we do what we do. It is so easy to settle into a working role in an industrial or health-care setting and, after a number of years, cease to question practices and working patterns. We fall into the 'we have always done it this way' syndrome. A well-conducted appraisal interview should provide a forum for the manager and the worker to look critically, yet objectively, at working roles, question established practices and seek alternative approaches which may be more effective.

Performance appraisal systems in many guises have been active for a long time and they continue to grow. The civil service and armed forces recognized their potential value many years ago and have pioneered new approaches which meet their specific needs. All organizations and services using a system do, of course, need to guard against the dangerous pitfall of managers paying lip-service to their scheme and failing to use it as a dynamic framework which responds to changing management needs.

GOOD MANAGEMENT PRACTICE

The manager has a responsibility for ensuring that the organization offers a framework within which the individual worker can develop and make a full contribution. Policies should positively encourage the development of:

● understanding and mutual trust through the establishment of effective channels of communication between workers at all levels;
● the maximum possible degree of delegation with accountability and management control;
● clear job descriptions defining not only the main functions but also the line communication and liaison links previously agreed with all the people concerned;
● an acceptance of the importance of training people for the jobs they are doing and preparing them for the future;
● flexible in-service education and training facilities geared to meet expressed needs as they arise.

Where these conditions exist, staff appraisal will make it possible for an objective, mutually agreed assessment to be made concerning:

- An individual's work performance, in terms of:
  areas of strength and weakness;
  areas of difficulty and frustration;
  future potential and ambitions;
  the kind of help needed now and in the future.
- The effectiveness of current management systems and organizational policies.
- The extent to which previously agreed aims and objectives have been reached and the setting of further aims to be achieved within an agreed period.

APPRAISAL SYSTEMS IN NURSING

The nursing profession prior to the 1970s had a reputation for failing to observe any ongoing appraisal system for its members once training was completed. In reality, it must be stated, however, that it was no worse than other disciplines within the health service. Sadly, the need for effective appraisal on a regular basis was ignored.

I recall an episode in my own working life which gave me a jolt. During a period as a senior nurse manager in the south of England, a well-respected paediatric ward sister retired from the hospital after twenty years' outstanding service in the same ward area. We organized the usual farewell tea party and presentation of gifts which was a pleasant occasion. The hospital paediatrician (who had worked closely with the sister during her long service) gave an informal speech, during which he expressed great admiration for the sister's contribution to the hospital. Other senior members of staff paid their tributes to the lady in glowing terms which were obviously fully justified. At the end of the day, the retiring sister came to the nursing office to say her final goodbye before actually leaving. She expressed her thanks for the party and gifts and was obviously moved and grateful for the warm praise of her colleagues. I remember her saying simply 'It was so kind of everyone to say such nice things about my work. I wish though that someone had told me during my twenty years on the ward that I was doing a good job – it would have helped a lot in difficult times.' It is rather sad that one had to wait for retirement to receive recognition and appreciation. One hopes that it could not happen today.

In 1977, the National Nursing Staff Committee (NNSC) issued a comprehensive report on staff appraisal for the hospital nursing service (DHSS, 1977). This followed a report produced earlier which introduced the concept of appraisal for nurses (DHSS, 1971). Also in 1971, some local government authorities had recommended an appraisal system for community nurses.

The NNSC system for nursing staff appraisal – which was based on extensive fieldwork and research – is still in use in many health authorities, but in some it has been modified or replaced altogether by a newer system, often referred to as performance review. These changes will be discussed later. Whatever system is in operation it is likely to have certain aims and be based on common principles.

Aims and principles of an appraisal system

● The prime objective is to improve performance with the ultimate aim of improving the effectiveness of the nursing service. To this end, the role of appraisal is seen to be:

to increase the contribution of individual nurses in their current job;
to develop the potential abilities to meet the need of the service in the future.

● The system should include a regular written appraisal of performance accompanied by an appraisal interview. (This takes place annually in the NNSC system, using the standard form shown in Appendix A.) Newly qualified staff would normally have their first appraisal after a shorter period of time, for example after six-months service. Notice of when the appraisal is to take place should be given and the nurse concerned should be reassured of the purpose of the meeting.

● It can be helpful for both appraisers and those countersigning the appraisal to receive guidance notes; these are an integral part of the NNSC system. In addition, it is important that both interviewees and interviewers prepare for the event. This can be aided by the completion of standard forms, examples of which are shown in Appendix B.

● The written appraisal and appraisal interview will normally be completed by the nurse to whom the appraised is directly accountable. At the interview, the nurse should be given the opportunity to discuss her progress and encouraged to talk freely about the way she sees the job, any difficulties she encounters and ways in which she might be helped to do it in a more effective manner. Her ambitions and inclinations should be discussed together with any further training or broadening of experience which might help her to achieve her aims. A constructive discussion will not only help the nurse in her work but will also help to improve the effectiveness of the organization as a whole. It must be recognized clearly, however, that this interview does, in no way, reduce the manager's responsibility for day-to-day counselling and advice, nor should it be used as part of any disciplinary procedure.

• A 'Development Action Plan' should be agreed between the appraiser and the appraisee. This plan is a simple statement in writing of objectives agreed between a senior nurse and her member of staff for the development of the latter. 'Development' includes the development of clinical, management or personal skills. It is important that the plan should be practicable, concentrating on one or two areas which call for some extra effort or an improvement in methods of working. The success of such plans will sometimes involve the help of nurses more senior to the parties to the agreement. Copies of the completed development action plan should be retained by the appraiser and the appraisee to assist in the monitoring of the plan.

• Self-appraisal can form an important part of the system since it shifts the emphasis away from an appraisal based solely on the views of the manager. One approach which has found support is to invite the appraisee to complete the form in pencil before the appraisal interview. In any case, provision should be made for the appraisee to sign and indicate that she has seen the assessment of her performance and has discussed it at the appraisal interview. She should also be able to add her own remarks.

• There should be a secure system for the storage of appraisal information but it should be made available to those senior nurses who need to follow up training recommendations. It was originally recommended that appraisal forms should be retained for five years and then destroyed, but health authorities should have their own policies relating to the retention of forms, usage of and access to information.

In conclusion, any appraisal or performance review system will only function if both appraisers and appraisees understand fully the principles to be followed. All appraisers should receive appropriate training in all aspects of the scheme, and each authority should review the policy for, and operation of, its scheme regularly.

The appraisal interview – the appraiser's role

This is the focal point of any appraisal scheme. The degree of skill and understanding with which it is conducted will certainly determine the success or failure of the total exercise. Equally, if badly conducted, it will adversely affect the working relationships between the manager and the appraisee. The experienced senior nurse conducting the interview should be confident and fully conversant with the range of skills required for a face-to-face interview.

There are a number of key points which the appraiser will wish to consider before the interview:

- Preparation should be thorough. Ensure that adequate notice is given. Study previous appraisals and development action plans.
- Complete the interviewer's preparation form (Appendix B) and plan a structure for the interview. Complete the appraisal form (in pencil or otherwise).
- Study the job description of the nurse to be appraised. Does this still accurately reflect the job which is being undertaken?
- Identify any personal prejudices or lack of understanding which may detract from an objective assessment of the appraisee's performance.

The interviewer must be prepared to look critically at her own perform-ance within the organization and how her management style affects colleagues and junior staff. There may well be occasions during an appraisal interview when the appraiser recognizes a failure on her part to support or guide staff. There are many important points which add up to an effective interview; one which merits particular attention is the need for the interviewer (or appraiser) to learn to listen closely to what is said and not said. Give the appraisee every opportunity to 'think out loud' without any fear of censure.

The 'dos and don'ts' for appraisers listed in Table 5.1 may be helpful.

Advice for the appraisee

The manager has a responsibility to assist the appraisee to prepare for the appraisal interview. We should not underestimate the concern and apprehension which the pending interview can arouse.

It might be helpful if the manager spent a short time with the nurse to be appraised about a week before the actual interview. The appraisee could be encouraged to prepare for the interview. The following points should be considered:

- Personal perception of performance since the last interview including accomplishments and difficulties encountered.

Table 5.1   Suggestions for appraisers

Do	Don't
Be prepared – make sure you have all the relevant information to hand.	Allow any interruptions during the interview.
Put the nurse at ease when she comes in by using normal social courtesies.	Allow yourself to be flustered or start fidgeting with objects on the table.
Be at ease yourself – be patient and unhurried.	Tell her 'Your trouble is . . .'.
Get the nurse to volunteer her own limitations.	Concentrate on personality traits.
	Try to cover everything.
Limit yourself to two or three important weaknesses and strengths.	Assume you know all about every incident discussed.
Give the nurse a proper chance to explain her points.	Give the nurse a false impression of your judgement of her by only discussing weaknesses.
Make sure good points are discussed and reinforced.	Shirk discussing weak areas.
Make sure needs/weaknesses are discussed.	Ask questions which can be answered by 'yes' or 'no'. Ask questions which give away the desired answer.
Ask 'open-ended questions' – 'Tell me about . . .'.	Give an excuse in the question e.g. 'You didn't do . . . because you were doing . . .'.
Ask neutral questions aimed at establishing fact.	
Keep control of the interview without being too inflexible.	Allow the nurse to dictate the course of the interview.
Establish practical objectives – if possible suggested by the nurse.	Force your own ideas on an unwilling receiver.
Encourage the nurse to develop herself.	Show impatience or boredom.
Be alert and interested throughout the interview.	Forget to summarize at the end of the interview.
Summarize what you have agreed and bring the interview to a 'natural' conclusion – give the nurse the opportunity to raise anything you have not discussed.	
Agree on an 'Action Plan' for the future.	

- Identify the most important activities in present job.
- Does the job fully utilize skills, training, knowledge and interests? If not, how could the job be changed in order to accomplish this?
- Whether there are weaknesses in present performance and how they might be overcome.
- Future aspirations? Is additional experience or further training needed in order to attain them?
- Are there any aspects of the organization one would change if given the authority?

Appraisal must be seen by both management and staff as a natural follow-up of day-to-day discussions and on-the-job guidance. It must never be allowed to degenerate into a meaningless ritual carried out by the manager without any positive participation from the appraisee.

TRAINING FOR APPRAISAL AND PERFORMANCE REVIEW

We have already referred to the principle that all managers undertaking the appraisal and interviewing role require training and support. In the past, many books on staff appraisal ended with a description of the actual process and failed to address the issue of preparing staff to conduct the system. The key to any successful training programme must be practice under guidance – improvement in interviewing ability comes only with practice.

The format for any agreed training programmes will obviously depend on the resources available. Experience in many health authorities, however, has shown clearly that there must be an ongoing programme using a range of training techniques. Ideally, there should be a designated senior nurse or training officer within each district who will have a co-ordinating role for the programme. Sessions in all induction courses for newly appointed nursing staff, together with monthly workshops, could provide a framework to ensure that all staff have the opportunity of participating. Sessions should include:

- discussion on principles of appraisal
- video films
- demonstration role play
- practice interviews
- practice with completion of appraisal forms.

The Industrial Society in London has pioneered a successful formula for introductory and advanced training modules in appraisal. Over the past five years, a number of first-class video training films and training kits have also become available. These films and kits can play a useful part in demonstrating the principles of appraisal and performance review systems. Staff can be assured that the system is simple and need not cause apprehension or undue concern.

Some considerations

A number of questions frequently recur in appraisal training sessions and the trainer would be wise to give them some thought beforehand if he is to deal with them effectively. There are many myths and misconceptions relating to appraisal schemes and therefore the organization or hospital group should have a firm philosophy and policy which covers all aspects of the scheme. It is well to start any training session for nurses with the unequivocable statement that *a good appraisal scheme will improve patient care* at all levels by ensuring the professional and personal development of nurses.

- *Is an appraisal scheme cost-effective?* This is a common question in the present NHS climate. The answer must be in the affirmative, although it is obviously difficult to quantify savings. We need, however, to remind ourselves simply that nurses form the major portion of the NHS workforce and much effort and expense goes into the selection and appointment of senior nurses. It must surely be imperative that we develop these nurses to their full potential. An appraisal scheme is one means of ensuring this development.
- *Where does the appraisal scheme start?* If the scheme is to be seen as important, it should start at the top and work downwards. The Chief Nurse (or Senior Nurse to the authority) must be seen to be personally involved in the scheme if it is to have full credibility. Starting at the top has the additional advantage that appraisers will normally have been appraised and this is a salutary experience which is likely to lead to improved interviewing skills.
- *Personality or performance – which do we appraise?* This is a fair question which must be addressed honestly. There is a strong emphasis on performance review in appraisal interviews. Can one assess the performance in isolation? It is recognized that it is extremely difficult to modify an individual's personality and yet there are occasions when the appraiser must say 'unless you change your style of dealing with

staff you will never achieve objectives'. It is not easy to ignore personality traits but the appraisee must be assured that the appraiser is making a real effort to review the level of working performance and overall effectiveness within the team.

● *Will appraisals be used for reference purposes?* It has been recommended that the appraisal should not be used for references because this may detract from the value of the interview and encouragement of open discussion. Some managers, however, feel that it is appropriate to study the appraisals completed (with overall gradings for performance) before actually completing a reference. It would obviously be quite improper to submit copies of completed appraisal forms to any prospective employer.

RECENT DEVELOPMENTS IN APPRAISAL AND PERFORMANCE REVIEW

The National Health Service structure, organization and philosophy have been undergoing dramatic changes in the past ten years. The concept of 'general management', as part of the Griffiths Report proposals, has acted as a stimulus to health authorities to reassess appraisal and performance monitoring systems.

Several health authorities have already replaced the NNSC staff appraisal system, or are in the position of developing a different system for the review of performance of staff. Individual Performance Review (IPR) is now operating quite widely at general manager level and there are signs that in some health authorities such a system is gradually being developed for use with all disciplines and at all levels. The emphasis in IPR is not just on performance and efficiency but also on individual development. It usually includes a number of factors:

● objectives are agreed;
● the individual's strengths and weaknesses are examined;
● the career aspirations are explored;
● a personal development plan which identifies training needs is drawn up;
● agreement on action is reached and a contract is made between the individual and the manager.

The rating of performance against agreed objectives, and the matching of five bands or levels of performance to different levels of bonus (performance-related pay) is a feature of some IPRs. However, other performance review systems are excluding rating and are not related to pay. (See Millar, 1988, for a discussion of performance-related pay.)

In addition to appraisal systems which focus on the manager's review of a subordinate's performance, there is also an increased use of peer review. This entails a nurse judging the work of her peers as well as being judged herself by them. It can work well alongside a staff appraisal scheme, but it also has some advantages over the latter. For example, the need in peer review to assess personal performance as well as that of others can be very beneficial, and helps to ensure that a two-way process occurs. In the USA, peer review systems are strongly linked with quality measurement, something that is only beginning to occur in the UK. (For an interesting discussion of peer review, see Wainwright, 1987.)

There is no perfect appraisal or performance review system and any organization must monitor its own and be prepared to adapt to changing needs. However, there is a need to move right away from 'the widely held concept of staff appraisal as a judgemental, retrospective process, where the nurse is "reported" on by her senior officer and in which she takes a purely passive role'. This was a conclusion of a major research project on nursing staff appraisal in the health service, commissioned from the Polytechnic of Central London in the early 1970s (Jones and Rogers, 1971). Although this research played a key role in setting parameters for guidance on the introduction of the NNSC scheme, an element of this problem still appears to exist today. One way of trying to overcome this concern is for the appraisal of individuals to be much more closely linked with the needs of the organization.

THE RELATIONSHIP BETWEEN INDIVIDUAL PERFORMANCE REVIEW AND QUALITY OF CARE

In the past there has been little emphasis in the NHS on the relationship between the appraisal of individuals and the development of the organization – in this instance the improvement of standards of care for patients and the monitoring of those standards. Now, in line with many of the major industrial and commercial organizations such as ICI, Shell, the major banks and several building societies, there is much more attention to this and a great deal is heard about quality assurance and methods of measuring quality.

Quality assurance

Quality assurance programmes are now an integral component of the strategy for every health authority in the United Kingdom. Nurses at all levels, in hospital and community settings, will be expected to play a full part in these exercises. General managers are charged with responsibility for ensuring that there is an ongoing system for developing, implementing and maintaining an effective pattern of QA activity. It has been suggested that this move is long overdue within the NHS where we have rarely defined in measurable terms what we sought to achieve.

A quality assurance programme can be described as a process whereby standards of care are continuously, objectively monitored and measured. The outcomes are then assessed against pre-established criteria and corrective action taken, when indicated. To understand the principles behind quality assurance one can usefully look at its history and development – mainly in the USA. American regulatory bodies have introduced guidelines for different aspects of the quality of health care. In the early 1960s, the American Nurses' Association outlined a model for the provision, evaluation and improvement of patient care. The Joint Commission on Accreditation of Hospitals (JCAH) in 1975 increased the number of multidisciplinary audits required for hospitals.

Although QA programmes in the USA have taken on a formal structure to satisfy outside agencies, it must be recognized that considerable progress had been made prior to the mandatory 'hospital accreditation system'.

Accreditation is a system whereby teams of doctor, administrator and nurse visit the hospital which seeks to be accredited. The team carries out a full survey based on questions, observation and interviews over three or four days. Recommendations for improvement are often made. The team may recommend that the hospital be accredited or, alternatively, suggest changes which must be made before accreditation is granted. As it is financially highly desirable to be an accredited institution most hospitals will do whatever is required.

Over the next years a number of patterns will be developed which seek to evaluate the outcomes and quality of care. These patterns will all emphasize the setting of clear objectives for the organization as a whole, specific disciplines and individuals. The objectives agreed for the individual will be an integral part of the annual staff appraisal and performance review exercise. This yearly review therefore will assume additional importance.

Assessing quality on the ward

One of the methods that is increasingly being used for judging quality of care on a ward is that known as MONITOR (Goldstone, Ball and Collier, 1984). (This is the UK form of the Rush Medicus Nursing Process

Methodology.) 'Monitor is proving popular with ward sisters and nurses because it shows exactly where care is failing and where improvements should be focused. It is popular with managers because it indicates which wards may be failing and why' (Slack, 1985).

The system allows the ward manager to describe the acuity (dependency) of each patient, the workload, the manpower required to achieve a prearranged level of quality and the appropriate staff mix. As such it can be a very powerful tool for the sister or charge nurse because it provides an objective assessment or diagnosis of what is actually happening on a ward, and can demonstrate that change is required and the nature of that change. It strengthens the ward manager's position since 'the demands made by the ward sister or charge nurse cannot be disregarded unless a lower measured standard is agreed. One manager has described the experience as 'holding a tiger by the tail' (Birch, 1986).

It has been claimed that the implementation of MONITOR in a ward can have many beneficial spin-offs such as the identification of training needs, the development of better ways of organizing the nursing care and the improvement of patient information. In addition, 'nurses frequently report improved confidence in their work after being "Monitored"; and the concept and practice of practical quality assurance seem to have arrived through the medium of Monitor' (Goldstone, 1987). Thus it can be seen that there are considerable potential links between an appraisal or performance review system, which also seeks to achieve some of these aims, and a system designed to assess systematically the 'performance' of a ward or other clinical setting. (For an interesting discussion of MONITOR and its use in nursing, see Goldstone, 1987.)

As part of this increasing emphasis on quality, a number of strategies have been devised to help improve quality as well as to measure it. One such method is that of quality circles.

Quality circles
Quality circles (QCs) are small groups of staff, usually from the same ward, unit or work area, which meet voluntarily and regularly to identify and solve their own work-related problems. The group has a leader plus a facilitator and reports its conclusions to the managers who decide on what action is to be taken. Sometimes the group has sufficient power and authority to take the action itself. It can be a very useful way of increasing commitment to total quality management and can have an effect on individual growth and commitment. Though rather more commonly found in industry and commerce, the idea has been taken up in some health authorities and, for example, in North Warwickshire Health

Authority, has resulted in significant improvements and savings in a unit for the handicapped.

Improvement in the quality of patient care has to be directly linked with improved performance amongst individuals. An appraisal or performance review system should provide a sound framework for monitoring performance, agreeing targets and assisting the individual to maximize her contribution.

To conclude, perhaps one of the biggest shifts that is required is a move away from the philosophy of external assessment (or 'judgment') which has often been a major feature of appraisal in the past to one of internal self reflection, assisted and supported by others.

> Self examination – if it is thorough enough – is nearly always the first step towards change. No one who learns to know himself remains just the same as before.
>
> (Thomas Mann)

ACKNOWLEDGEMENTS

I wish to acknowledge particularly the ideas obtained from *Staff Appraisal for Nurses* published by the Nursing Division of South West Metropolitan Regional Hospital Board (1973).

Sample forms in the Appendices are taken from the *Report of the National Staff Committee for Nurses and Midwives on NHS Staff Development and Performance Review* (1977).

REFERENCES AND SUGGESTIONS FOR FURTHER READING

Birch, J. (1986) Quality assurance, *Senior Nurse*, Vol.5, pp.20–1.

Department of Health and Social Security (1971) *Staff Appraisal in the Nursing Service*, DHSS, London.

Department of Health and Social Security (1977) *Report of the National Staff Committee for Nurses and Midwives on NHS Staff Development and Performance Review*, DHSS, London.

Drucker, P.F. (1971) *The Effective Executive*, Heinemann, London.

Goldstone, L. (1987) Monitor, in A. Pearson (ed.) *Nursing Quality Measurement*, Wiley, Chichester.

Goldstone, L., Ball, J. and Collier, M. (1984) *MONITOR: An Index of the Quality of Nursing Care for Acute Medical and Surgical Wards*, Newcastle-upon-Tyne Polytechnic Products Ltd.

Jones, D. and Rogers, A. (1971) *Nursing Staff Appraisal in the Health Service: A Study of the System*, Polytechnic of Central London.

Millar, B. (1988) Pay plans aims to reward increased responsibility, *The Health Service Journal*, Vol. 98, no. 5082, p. 8.
Slack, W.P. (1985) Standards of care, *Nursing Times*, 29 May, pp. 28–32.
Wainwright, P. (1987) Peer review, in A. Pearson (ed.) *Nursing Quality Measurement*, Wiley, Chichester.

Appendix A

FORM FOR COMPLETION BY INTERVIEWERS

This form has been designed on the assumption that good nursing care involves all or most of the aspects of performance set out below. Please read the notes for guidance of appraisers and countersigners before completing the appraisal and throughout its completion.

Aspects of performance

In this part of the form you consider the skills required to carry out the duties as described. You should make as much use as possible of the spaces for comment so as to provide as full a picture as possible. Use the 'I' (importance) column to show for each aspect of performance whether it is high (H), medium (M) or low (L).

ASPECT	I	A	B	C	D	E	F	COMMENT

1. Organization and management of work

2. Supervision of staff and leadership

3. Relationships:
   a. With patients/clients, their relatives etc.
   b. With immediate colleagues, administrative, ancillary and other groups of staff
   c. With Social Services Department, schools and supportive agencies
   d. With nursing management
   e. With learners, visiting lecturers and other visitors.

4. Ability to communicate:
   a. orally
   b. in writing.

ASPECT	I	A	B	C	D	E	F	COMMENT

5. Teaching and training:
   a. Patients, their relatives etc.
      (e.g. health education)
   b. Qualified staff (e.g. in ongoing
      on-the-job development)
   c. On-the-job training of
      students, pupils etc.
   d. Education of students/pupils
      in formal and informal settings

6. Ability to contribute/develop/
   carry out new ideas and methods

7. Analysis of problems, their
   solution, and decision making

8. Other relevant skills not covered
   above
   a.

   b.

Summary of performance overall – including comments on general care of patients and clients in suitable cases

Training needs and development of potential

1. Has the appraised been the subject of any form of development action during the past year? If so, please comment giving, if possible, an assessment of any effect on performance/confidence.

2. Would he/she benefit from and be suitable for any form of development action during the coming year? If so, please specify: state briefly the aim of the action proposed and complete a Development Action Plan form, copies of which should be held by those principally concerned.

3. Does the appraised have any special aptitudes or inclinations? Could these be better used than at present for the benefit of the Service and the nurse himself/herself? If so, please give your recommendations.

4. To what extent are your comments based on personal knowledge of the nurse and his/her work?

Signature of Appraiser...........................Grade...........................Date....

Remarks of countersigning nurse

1. Is the appraised satisfied that this appraisal is both accurate and fair? Yes/No.

2. If the answer to 1. is 'No', what action is called for?

3. I note the assessment made above and the Development Action Plan. I have the following additional comments to make, all of which I have discussed with the nurse and his/her appraiser:

4. (To be completed where no Development Action is proposed.) I have the following comments to make in respect of the appraisee's training and development needs:

5. To what extent are your comments based on personal knowledge of the nurse and her work?

Signature of countersigning nurse..............Grade..........................Date....

Remarks (if any) and signature of appraised

I have seen the above assessment of my performance and have discussed it at an appraised interview. I would like to add the following remarks:

Signature of appraised..Date....

Appendix B

INTERVIEWER'S PREPARATION FORM

1. You will shortly be giving an appraisal interview to M...............................
a member of your staff, at which his/her performance of his/her duties over the past year and in the coming year will be discussed.

2. You should have received some training in the techniques of interviewing before you conduct an appraisal interview. These notes are not intended as a substitute for such training; they are meant to serve simply as a reminder of the main points to be borne in mind in preparing for and conducting an interview.

3. The purpose of the interview is to provide an occasion for a two way exchange of views at which the appraisee should be given full opportunity to discuss his/her job, the way it is organized, how he/she thinks the quality of his/her contribution might be improved, and so on. If he/she has agreed to complete an interview preparation form, the foundation of a well planned interview will have been laid. If he/she has not completed one you might find it helpful to proceed along the lines of the agenda set out below which is, of course, made up from the main headings of the interview preparation form. On the other hand, it should be recognized that there is no precisely correct way to conduct an appraisal interview and you may wish or find it necessary to vary the agenda. Whatever form the interview takes the appraisee should come away from it quite

clear as to where he/she stands and about what he/she needs to do to achieve any personal objectives which may have been agreed for the coming year.

4. Whichever method you adopt, however, it is important that you should get off on the right footing by having paid attention to one or two matters of detail as follows:

a. Give as much notice as possible (and normally not less than 3 days). Arrange the appointment at a mutually satisfactory date and time if at all possible.

b. Ask the nurse to complete an interview preparation form or at least think about the headings on the form.

c. Allow adequate time for the interview (which may vary according to circumstances and the personalities involved).

d. Ensure complete privacy and freedom from telephones and bleeps etc.

e. Finally, remember that although there are no simple rules for establishing rapport at interviews most people will respond to some evidence that the interviewer has a genuine concern for them as individual human beings and that he/she does not regard them merely as members of staff.

Agenda

The past year's work.
Obstacles encountered by appraisee.
Appraisee's suggestions for improvement of his/her job performance.
Appraisee's personal development programme.
Appraisee's career.
Any other points.

INTERVIEWEE'S PREPARATION FORM

1. You will shortly be invited to an appraisal interview at which you will be able to discuss your work during the past year and in the coming year. You will also have the opportunity to discuss any other matter on which you feel you need help or advice in order that you may obtain greater satisfaction from your work and develop your potential to the full.

2. To help you and the interviewer obtain the most benefit from the interview you are asked to complete this form. It is your own personal form which you may or may not show to the interviewer as you wish. Some staff may be asked to complete their own appraisal form in pencil as part of a self-assessment, in which case they may not need to complete this form in full.

3. When the interview is over you can decide whether you wish to keep or destroy this form or whether you would like to have it filed with your completed appraisal.

Key tasks

Set down here a brief list of what you consider to be the key tasks or responsibilities in your job. Although you will have been (or will be) asked to agree a list

of key tasks, you may like to set these out again on this form for ease of reference during the interview and/or for your personal retention.
1.

2.

3.

4.

5.

6.

The past year's work
What have you done best, or with greatest satisfaction? (Think of, for example: clinical performance; organization and management; relationships with patients' relatives and visitors; liaison with other staff; supervision; teaching and training; or any other contributions you may have made to the benefit of the patient/client).

Obstacles
Were there any obstacles which hindered you from accomplishing what you would have wished? Are they likely to recur?

Improvement
To make your job performance better what changes might be made by:
a. Your immediate superior or higher management?
b. Yourself?
c. Anyone else?

Development programme for the coming year
Assuming that development plans for the next year are practicable, in what way do you think you could best demonstrate your ability to improve on acknowledged good performance or overcome any weaknesses?

Career
What do you hope to be doing in, say, 3 years' time? And how do you see your career developing? In this connection, is there any question you wish to ask or anything you wish to mention at the interview? (You will, of course, appreciate that the interviewer cannot make promises but may nevertheless be able to help with advice.)

NOTE

The Appendices give only sample parts of the NHS Staff Development and Performance Review forms to show the approach adopted.

In order to use this system properly reference would need to be made to the complete forms, which include guidance notes.

6. Communication Skills

Joanna Gray

INTRODUCTION

There are certain problematical and fundamental questions to be addressed before it is possible to determine the place and prominence of communication skills in the professional development of nurses. Given that the basis of any successful interaction is mutual understanding, it is essential to establish an agreement of terminology and urgency. The five inherent questions are:

- *What* is understood by 'communication skills'?
- *Why* should it be necessary to include such training in the professional development of nurses?
- *Whether* it is possible to develop these skills and measure or assess development.
- *How* can the development of these skills be facilitated?
- *Which* specific interpersonal skills should take precedence in professional development?

This chapter will consider the questions and attempt to provide answers based on the author's experience of practical and documented development sessions. The majority of these sessions were included in the London Postgraduate Teaching Hospitals Scheme, which, from its inception, placed great emphasis on the inclusion of communication skills training.

WHAT IS UNDERSTOOD BY 'COMMUNICATION SKILLS'?

In these days of jargon and journalese, it is particularly important to establish that there are common referential terms and to de-mystify the terminology and the process. Communication, whether conscious or unconscious, occurs whenever people come together. It is impossible *not* to communicate. Experienced nurses are well aware that the most withdrawn patient, the most compliant patient, the most aggressive patient is communicating something. The difficulty lies in whether or not the communication is received and interpreted accurately; whether the receiver appreciates the need to confirm the interpretation; and whether the response is appropriate to the stimulus. The skills involved are *interpersonal* and should be narrowed down to this definition. Training experience should be concentrated on nurses communicating with patients, relatives and colleagues in a caring and concerned capacity.

WHY SHOULD IT BE NECESSARY TO INCLUDE SUCH SKILLS TRAINING IN THE PROFESSIONAL DEVELOPMENT OF NURSES?

Published research has shown that nurses' interpersonal skills have not been adequate to satisfy patients' needs. Recent research goes back to Ashworth (1981), Bridge and Macleod Clark (1981), and Wilson-Barnett (1983). More recent research by Faulkner (1985) states that there has been a considerable shift towards accepting the need for communication and counselling skills in nursing. She goes on to say that there is much research which shows that nurses do not present the interpersonal skills needed by patients. Should any doubts remain as to researched evidence, the Reports of the Health Service Commissioner provide a rich and useful source of documented investigation. Most of the above mentioned research is concerned with acute care, but such care does not describe the boundaries of the nursing profession nor does it represent membership of the Postgraduate Teaching Hospitals Scheme. Jean McIntosh (1981) has given an eloquent description of the importance of interpersonal skills and their relationship to care in the community. McIntosh uses the words 'role', 'status' and 'balance' as involved in the ambivalent position of the district nurse. She poses questions directly relevant to the rationale of any attempt to develop nurses' interpersonal skills. For example:

● If nurses take the role of 'hostess' in a ward and the different role of 'guest' in the home, does this affect the nature of communication in the two settings?
● How does adopting either of these two roles affect a particular interaction or a longer term relationship?
● How do nurses and clients use 'tactics' to cope, influence, persuade or manipulate? How aware are they that such 'tactics' are being used?

The words 'role', 'status' and 'balance' are key words and help to explain why professional development in interpersonal skills is valued. The historical perception, professional and public, of a nurse as 'the lady with the lamp', instantly responding to medical orders, neatly uniformed and crisply coping without visible emotion, has mitigated against the use and development of inherent interpersonal skills. How can you care if you are only meant to cure?

Vestiges of this particular role perception still linger, for example in the transition from student nurse to staff nurse; from staff nurse to sister/charge nurse. In fact, the ward sister lives a multiplicity of professional roles. Referring again to McIntosh's study of role, status and balance, it is important to examine the implications for personal and professional development and training. Such examination shows that fulfilment of expectations will require sensitive and sophisticated inter-personal skills. Table 6.1 presents an analysis of some of these skills.

It should no longer be necessary to ask *why* ward sisters and charge nurses need support and development in the area of interpersonal skills. Nursing, if it is to be a profession, requires communication skills beyond those of the layman. And nurse managers, if they are to fulfil the role, require opportunities for training, stimulus, sharing, information and experiential development. If these opportunities are not provided, human potential will be wasted and the ultimate loss will be a loss of care and caring.

Table 6.1   Roles and interpersonal skills

Roles	Skills

Clinician
Teacher
Negotiator
Interpreter
Manager
Counsellor
Policy-maker
	Observation
	Explanation
	Choice of appropriate language
	Use of non-verbal skills
	Ability to suspend judgement
	Awareness of questioning skills and
	   their aims
	Active listening with appropriate
	   feedback
	Ability to use silence
	Self-awareness
	Ability to distinguish between
	   assertion and aggression

Status	**Skills**
Authority Accountability Responsibility	Stress management Self awareness Management of time Assertiveness Ability to clarify Listening skills
Balance	**Skills**

Discussing rather than demanding
Helping to do rather than doing to
Listening with rather than listening to
Counselling rather than
   reprimanding
Developing staff rather than
   'containing' them
Exploiting change rather than
   resisting it
	All the interpersonal skills previously
	   mentioned as well as specific
	   training in law, labour relations,
	   staff appraisal, etc.

IS IT POSSIBLE TO TEACH OR DEVELOP INTERPERSONAL SKILLS?

Lathlean, in Chapter 10, makes many comments relevant to the issue, e.g.

● 'it is crucial to examine a situation from a number of perspectives,

including the experiences of participants' (see p. 161).
● 'From the evaluation questionnaires, the answers to questions about the most and least beneficial subjects were interesting. In an analysis of responses gained from the first series of courses, there was considerable common ground in the subjects chosen as most beneficial with six subjects being listed by over half of all respondents. These were communications, research, counselling, assertiveness training, legal aspects and discipline and grievance. This concurs with the findings of Lathlean and Farnish, 1984, in their evaluation of a ward sister training scheme, where the three most frequently mentioned topics of most benefit were research, counselling and communications (see p. 167).

Managers were asked to comment on developments and a common theme throughout their replies was that of improved communication skills and a better approach to staff.

In the author's experience, participants have found interpersonal skills sessions to be 'thought-provoking, unsettling, stimulating, worrying, supportive'. As the chief objective of two four-hour sessions was to increase awareness, participants' evaluation of their feelings was crucial. It is impossible to provide scientifically supported evidence that training in interpersonal skills produces immediate, measurable results. Indeed, any such results would be open to question as attitudes are slow and difficult to change. What is most relevant is that ward sisters and charge nurses themselves have valued the opportunity to examine their own interpersonal skills.

HOW CAN SKILLS DEVELOPMENT AND AWARENESS BE FACILITATED?

Before experienced nurses can be asked to undertake potentially threatening activities, the 'atmosphere of harmony' suggested by Verena Tschudin (1985) must be created. Beryl Heather in a booklet produced by the FPA Education Unit (1984) advises us that the most effective way to give relevant information and to develop awareness and skills is by using group methods which encourage participation and sharing of experiences in a comfortable atmosphere. Philip Burnard (1985) emphasizes the necessity of self-awareness training in the caring professions. Some of his very telling comments are:

If we are unaware and blind to ourselves, then we will remain blind to others.

The process begins with me. I must first examine myself.

Unfortunately, what often happens is that nurses notice what is happening around them – to patients, to colleagues or to the environment – but pay little attention to what happens to themselves.

Self-awareness is neither easy nor pain-free, but it is an essential beginning to any development of interpersonal skills. These skills are often recognized in small groups within a 'safe' environment. To quote LaMonica and Karshmer (1978), 'The core of the helping process is interpersonal. Groups are inherently interpersonal. Group training in interpersonal functioning is the preferred mode of learning interpersonal skills. Training in interpersonal skills is the crux of coping with life.'

In order to determine a philosophy and methodology, the author has found it useful to isolate certain key words and phrases. These will serve as a painful reminder when a traditional approach tends to impinge. Such phrases as

- relevant information,
- awareness and skills,
- shared experience,
- examine yourself and pay attention to what is happening,
- role, status and balance,
- systematic thought and particular incident analysis,
- group interpersonal functioning,

should be helpful, not only for the facilitator but for the participants as well.

It is a truism to state that individuals learn and develop in individual ways. One of the anomalies in nurse education, however, is that individual learning processes have not been recognized. There has been a traditional right or wrong, correct or incorrect procedural approach to nurse training. This approach may be suitable for clinical procedures but it tends to establish a medical model of illness rather than the concept of the person. Interactions cannot be charted and measured in the same way that clinical observations are.

This awareness of traditional approaches to teaching and learning as contrasted with the clinical experience and real interaction with patients, relatives and colleagues helps to explain the suspicion, nervousness and perhaps cynicism which ward and community managers may feel when presented with the prospect of developing communication skills. So ward and community managers will vary enormously in their expectations of continuing development. Expectations will probably be based on previous experience; individual learning styles; shared objectives with senior managers; opportunity to put experience into practice and acceptance of colleagues.

These variables imply certain general principles for the facilitation of interpersonal skills. The guidelines the author follows are these:

- Make no assumptions and feel the way carefully. This is a sensitive area.
- Find out 'where they are'. Elicit from and relate to participants' experience.
- Provide the theory of the communication process and the methods and tools of communication but vary the pace by giving lively examples and opportunity to put theory into practice through discussion and experiential activities.
- Develop from perceived problems into constructive change. For example, most people are poor listeners albeit unaware of this deficiency. Active listening skills can be developed by practice in total involvement, selective editing and check-back.
- Finish on a positive note. The group and individual members should feel optimistic and encouraged.

Table 6.2 Participative model of skills development

Facilitator's contributions:	
information	guidelines
freedom of expression	confidentiality
opportunities for interaction and problem-solving	

Participants' contributions:	
personal experience	involvement
knowledge	motivation
sharing of expertise	

WHICH SPECIFIC INTERPERSONAL SKILLS SHOULD TAKE PRECEDENCE IN PROFESSIONAL DEVELOPMENT?

Since the introduction of the nursing process and reinforced by the media and the increasing demands of the public, nurses have faced criticism as to their lack of skills. Much of this criticism is confused and unsubstantiated. Learned and acquired social skills are the foundation of professional skills but they are inadequate and sometimes inappropriate for the professional role.

Faulkner (1986) has commented on the significant differences between social and professional interaction, listing four main categories: skills, content, power and choice. To these categories the author, with suggestions from course participants, would add: purpose, outcome, environment and stress. As we examine the above categories, the *professional* skills of interaction will become obvious, particularly when we relate them to the needs of the patient/client and the particular difficulties and constraints. Burton (1985) claims that 'interpersonal skills are not an end, but a means to an end. The end is good interactions for the users of the service (patients or clients). Just what a good interaction is will depend upon the needs of the user, both at the moment a particular interaction takes place and within the longer-term development of that person.' Burton goes on to say that 'to happen effectively, interactions

(1) have actually to take place;
(2) have to be sustained for as long as necessary rather than being cut off prematurely;
(3) have to have an appropriate content.'

The following representation of patients' needs, nurses' skills and environmental constraints is intended to demonstrate a few of the complexities of professional interaction.

Background information

Jennifer Croft has recently been appointed to the post of sister on

Florence Ward, a medical ward in a busy inner city hospital. It is 10.00 a.m., Staff Nurse Ingram has reported sick, leaving the ward understaffed again with 1 staff nurse, 2 enrolled nurses and 2 second-year students. There are 19 patients, a few of whom are elderly and highly-dependent. The Consultant's Round is scheduled to begin at 10.30 a.m. The telephone has been ringing incessantly and the most recent call was answered by a student, who reported that 'a lady was being sent up from Casualty for observation'. Sister Croft would have liked to use this inadequate message as an opportunity for teaching; however, she was supervising the other student nurse. Enrolled Nurse Turner was asked to clarify the information and it developed that Mrs Frances Holmes, 66, had presented with severe vomiting. Casualty Staff Nurse had taken particulars and called for a porter.

Development

Mrs Holmes' needs	Sister Croft's interpersonal skills	Environmental constraints
• Physical comfort • Psychological reassurance • Confidence in the professional skills of the carers, the efficiency of the organization • Information about what was to happen and why	• Establishing rapport • Using non-verbal skills of touch and gaze • Respecting need for personal space • Sensitive questioning • Selective information giving	• Lack of information • Background noise • Interruptions • Confused priorities • Lack of privacy • Mrs Holmes' anxieties • Assumptions

Outcome

Fortunately for Mrs Holmes, Sister Croft's interpersonal and managerial skills helped to make a potentially 'difficult' patient into a relatively comfortable person.

Process

- When the porter arrived with Mrs Holmes, Sister Croft made sure that she and a student nurse were there to receive Mrs Holmes, thank the porter and enlist his help in settling her down.
- Sister gave Mrs Holmes only the most relevant information, concentrating on her physical comfort.
- Mrs Holmes appeared to be much relieved by Sister's reassuring interventions and by her calm, caring professional manner. After medication and a sleep, Sister, with the student nurse, asked Mrs Holmes a few more questions, explaining why the information was needed. As the questions were open-ended, Mrs Holmes volunteered a great deal of information, making it unnecessary to ask a barrage of distressing questions.
- While Sister Croft was talking to Mrs Holmes, she was careful to respect the patient's personal space, to sit in a position which made it possible to establish and maintain eye contact, to ensure as much privacy as possible and to listen with all her senses. Sister was careful to check back from time to time, to make sure that she had understood and to avoid assumptions. For example, it appeared that Mrs Holmes was anxious about 'her Joe'. She and Joe had both had some of that chicken. She did hope Joe wasn't feeling as ill as she was.
- Having learned that Joe was a toy poodle and Mrs Holmes's only companion, Sister promised to see that Joe was looked after and to let Mrs Holmes know how he was getting on. She took that opportunity to give Mrs Holmes information about procedures on Florence Ward and to answer the patient's questions about her condition.
- As Mrs Holmes seemed to be getting tired, Sister Croft made sure that she was comfortable, explained that she would be coming back from time to time, gave Mrs Holmes a gentle pat on the hand and went on to see other patients.

Analysis

Sister Croft's interaction with Mrs Holmes satisfies Burton's three conditions of effective interactions: initiation, maintenance of contact, and appropriate content. Sister Croft demonstrated the skills of:

- *awareness* of colleagues' and patients' needs;

● *decision-making*, in that she decided to maintain patient contact rather than be diverted by other concerns;
● *information-giving*, by realizing that a person in pain or discomfort cannot take in much information;
● *questioning* used purposefully and sensitively;
● *listening and check-back, non-verbal communication* through eye contact, proximity, body positioning and touch;
● and finally, Sister Croft avoided making assumptions and refused to be judgemental or de-valuing. As a result, trust and rapport were established.

CONCLUSION

The following are the priorities in interpersonal skills development:

● *Awareness*
of personal values, beliefs, prejudices, impact on others, behaviour, idiosyncrasies;
of cultural and regional differences, illness and pain as inhibitors, the institution as a de-personalizing environment, the tendency to categorize according to age, class, sex, etc., the patient/client as a person with a past and a future, colleagues as involved members of a caring unit;
of the dangers of making unchecked-out assumptions based on hearsay, ambiguous written 'information', appearance, accent, facial expression.
● *Training in behaviour*
interaction in pairs and small groups, listening for spoken and unspoken content, selective listening, reflecting and paraphrasing, use of non-verbal communication, dealing with verbal 'aggression'; experiencing a simulated patient situation; e.g. being talked down to and over, being asked intimate questions in public, lying half-dressed on a trolley, being ignored, being talked to in jargon or pseudo-scientific language, being given treatment or medication without information, having choice curtailed. The beginning of a true understanding and experience of empathy.
● *Transfer and consolidation*
through experience and discussion to self-analysis and positive programmes for change . . . to personal behaviour, professional role,

environmental improvements. Some of the encouraging comments are illustrated below:

Never again will I say love or ducks to a patient.

We all assumed he had dentures because he was seventy-two. Well, he didn't.

I'm now aware that when I'm under stress, I frown or scowl. That may explain why nurses and patients keep away from me.

English politeness conventions are not a part of my culture. I've always found it difficult to say 'please' and 'thank you' constantly. But if it makes such a difference, I'll make an effort.

I looked at the photograph on the lady's locker. The woman was so beautiful that I couldn't help exclaiming: 'Who in the world is that gorgeous creature?' The patient turned away and began to cry. In future, I'll try to think before I speak.

I've never understood why intelligent, educated people should behave so stupidly when they come into hospital. When I was doing that exercise, I began to realise that intelligence hasn't anything to do with it.

We all do and say these horrible things. We'd just better admit it and try not to.

The final comment sums up the purpose and value of interpersonal skills training. Nurses are *people*, dealing with more physical and emotional stress than most professionals. Therefore, they are fallible humans not 'angels' or robots. The most anyone can ask is that they are aware and willing to work towards constructive change and that they are given the opportunities to develop personally and professionally.

REFERENCES

Ashworth, P. (1981) Communicating with patients and relatives in the intensive care unit, in W. Bridge and J. Macleod Clark (eds) *Communication in Nursing Care*, pp. 63–83. HM & M, London.
Burnard, P. (1985) *Learning Human Skills: A Guide for Nurses*, pp. 1–28. Heinemann, London.
Burton, M. (1985) The environment, good interactions and interpersonal skills in nursing, Part II, in C. Kagan (ed.) *Interpersonal Skills in Nursing: Research and Applications*, pp. 65–76. Croom Helm, Kent.

Faulkner, A. (1985) The evaluation of teaching interpersonal skills to nurses, Part V. in C. Kagan (ed.) *Interpersonal Skills in Nursing: Research and Applications*, Croom Helm, Kent.

Faulkner, A. (1986) Talking to patients: making contact. *Nursing Times*, Vol. 82, no. 33.

Heather, B. (1984) *Sharing*, FPA Education Unit, London.

La Monica, E. L. and Karschmer, J. F. (1978) Empathy: educating nurses in professional practice, *Journal of Nursing Education*, Vol. 17, no. 2. Quoted in V. Tschudin (1985) *Beginning with Empathy*. Learning Resources Unit of the English National Board for Nursing, Midwifery and Health Visiting, Sheffield.

Macleod Clark, J. and Bridge, W. (eds.) (1981) *Communication in Nursing Care*, HM & M, London.

McIntosh, J. (1981) Communicating with patients in their own homes, in W. Bridge and J. Macleod Clark (eds) *Communication in Nursing Care*, pp. 99–115. HM & M, London.

Tschudin, V. (1985) *Beginning with Empathy*. Learning Resources Unit of the English National Board for Nursing, Midwifery and Health Visiting, Sheffield.

Wilson-Barnett (ed.) (1983) *Nursing Research: Ten Studies in Patient Care*, Wiley, Chichester.

7. Teaching and Learning

Robert Cooper

The role of the sister in relation to teaching and learning is an important one, since all grades of nurse need to learn at each stage. With this in mind, the ward sister has to consider her staff's learning needs from the perspective of the adult learner. Whilst this statement may seem rather obvious, if one is not aware that adult learners differ in many respects from school children, in just how they learn, then problems may arise during attempts at teaching. Indeed nursing tends to have the reputation of being rather maternalistic in its treatment of its younger members and, if this is actually the case, it could be counter productive in the teaching and learning environment.

If the sister wishes to maximize the benefits from the teaching of nursing in the ward, it may be useful for her to consider some of the main points relevant to adult learning.

THE ADULT LEARNER

It is very important to stimulate adult learners and to provide plenty of relevant activity. This forms an important part of the role of the sister. The motivation can be, initially, the ward sister's enthusiasm for the nursing on the ward, which hopefully transfers to those in the role of learner. Further motivation may arise when the learner strives to do well on a ward known for its high standard of nursing care. The activity can be closely controlled by the ward sister as she is usually the overall organizer of care.

Adult learners like to feel that what they are learning is going to be both useful and relevant (Rogers, 1977). This condition can be met very adequately when nursing skills are being taught on the ward. Knowledge of results is another aspect of adult learning that the sister should consider, as an adult learner is ever keen to know their stage of progress. This carries with it the possibility of telling someone that they are not, in fact, progressing at all and this is equally as important as telling someone they have made progress.

Reinforcement is a further aspect of adult learning worthy of attention, as the teacher needs to lead the learner on to identify what an adequate performance is. This is usually achieved by frequent practice which reinforces previously learned skills. There is evidence to suggest that in the area of manual skills, spaced practice may be better than concentrated practice, particularly in the early stages of skills acquisition. However, some adult learners prefer longer periods of practice as they find these more beneficial (Rogers, 1977).

The sister should also be aware that even older members of staff can learn to learn and that this ability to learn can be improved despite what they may infer to the contrary. However, they need understanding and help to build up their confidence as they may have been allowed to work on over the years with little or no thought having been given to their learning needs.

COMMENT ON THE PAST

It is generally considered that the teaching of students and other less experienced nurses should be part of the role of all registered nurses. Indeed the Halsbury Committee (1974) recognized the teaching role when deciding on increased remuneration for nurses. However, whether or not registered nurses actually engage in teaching, as a fully recognized and integrated part of what they do, is open to debate.

Revans (1964) surveyed sixteen wards in a general hospital, all of which were training areas for student nurses, and found that in ten of the wards, no time was spent on the activity of teaching nurses during the period of the survey, and in two wards 1.8 per cent and 2.2 per cent of the time, respectively, was devoted to this activity.

Nightingale (1882) stated that nurses must be taught to teach – she was particularly referring to the ward sister – but this recommendation does not seem to have been taken very seriously over the intervening century. This perhaps indicates that the profession does not have a strong teaching tradition in the area of clinical practice and that much of a nurse's skill may have been acquired by trial and error learning or 'sitting with Nellie' and only occasionally by structured one to one sessions.

Melia (1987) states that 'much of the on-the-job learning happens between learners, senior apprentices teaching junior apprentices . . .'. However, unless strong emphasis is given to the subjects of teaching and learning in the basic and post-basic nursing courses it is doubtful if teaching will figure very largely in the registered nurses' repertoire.

COMMENT ON THE PRESENT

There appear to be mixed views amongst registered nurses as to whether or not they have a clearly identified teaching role. Indeed it would seem that many registered nurses working in training areas do not actively engage in the teaching of student nurses, yet this is often not taken up by more senior nurses, including ward sisters. It may reflect how ward teaching is perceived by the profession and the inadequacy that many sisters feel about their own teaching abilities (Farnish, 1983).

However, the hard fact remains that student nurses spend two-thirds of their training time working alongside sisters and staff nurses and the remainder with tutorial staff. When one considers the power of role models on these, often impressionable, young learners, it may be reasonable to suggest that it is the present generation of sisters and staff nurses that are shaping tomorrow's nurses, a fact that is often insufficiently recognized and exploited.

Indeed, registered nurses do appear to be interested in the subject of teaching and learning as illustrated by a study that the author is presently conducting on continuing education for registered nurses. When staff nurses were asked to select from a list of twenty-three subjects, six subjects that they considered should be included in a post-basic management course for staff nurses, teaching and learning was the most frequently chosen of the twenty-three subjects by the one hundred and nine respondents. This finding has also been highlighted by the research of Lathlean, Bradley and Smith (1986) and Vaughan (1980). (It is also reinforced by the popularity in many English health authorities of the ENB 998 course on Teaching and Assessing.)

Despite the foregoing, and much other research which indicates that there are major deficiencies in the teaching and learning of nursing, the ward sister is in a potentially strong position to do much to improve the status of teaching and learning in the clinical area – not only in respect of student nurses, but for all nurses including herself.

SETTING THE SCENE

There is little doubt as to the influence of the ward sister in the day-to-day running of the ward and it is this influence that can be used to create a teaching and learning environment that works to the benefit of patients and nurses alike. Research has indicated (see for example, Marson, 1987) that both sisters and learners tend to associate teaching and learning with lecturing and listening but, in fact, significant learning is often self-initiated and arises from personal experience rather than didactic instruction. An important prerequisite to facilitating this kind of learning is an environment where teaching and learning are valued and one which has certain features and resources to promote such activities.

Promoting teaching and learning in the clinical setting

If a sister wants to develop her ward to promote both teaching and learning she should first consider the state of the interpersonal relationships between members of staff, because if there are high levels of tension between staff this can result in learners disliking the ward (Fretwell, 1982). This will inevitably have a negative effect on their ability to learn as well as that of the trained nurses. Thus in some instances improving relationships may be a primary task.

The next point to think of is the views of staff. Staff consultation should take place prior to any attempt to implement a teaching policy or plan. It is crucial that all staff are, at least to some extent, in favour of the idea. The sister should not be too surprised if some of her staff nurses appear hesitant or are at first hostile to the idea, as they may feel vulnerable in relation to their own knowledge base. Indeed it may be that the trained staff would benefit from having their own knowledge and skills updated first, and this could be an area where the use of self-study materials may be appropriate.

In this situation the sister should try to find out what her staff feel they need in the way of updating and development, and then steps could be taken to find suitable learning packages, books, other appropriate materials and ways of gaining the necessary skills and knowledge. With guidance from the sister the formation of a study group may be possible, thus enabling peer group learning, with the sister participating and co-ordinating where necessary. Another useful strategy can be the development of seminars or discussion groups where each member of nursing staff is in turn responsible for presenting a paper on a topic of his or her choice that they have researched and studied. However, whatever the methods used, it is important that what is learned within the group can be used to enhance the nursing care given to patients. In other words, the theory and practice must be two sides of the one coin and efforts made to avoid the school/ward division often experienced by student nurses (Melia, 1987).

Peer-group learning can have a considerable effect not only on those taking part but also on more junior staff who see their role models actively engaged in studying the art of nursing as an integral part of their job. Also, learning by observing other more experienced nurses is known to be an important facet in clinical settings. This can be greatly enhanced by ensuring that the opportunities are there to learn from others, that the behaviour is worth observation (to avoid repeating someone else's bad practice) and that there is the chance to discuss what is observed.

It is important for the sister to give the creation of a good learning environment the priority it deserves and not allow it to be sacrificed to other pressures which may attempt to compete. It is at times like these when the sister will be required to support and even defend her system. She must keep staff motivated and interested, and she must guard against using the acquisition of knowledge as a competition as this may only serve to increase staff anxiety. She must encourage staff to share nursing knowledge with each other in the interests of patient care. This sharing requires trust between members of staff – a characteristic of a profession.

The school of nursing can be of considerable help here to provide information on what is available in terms of teaching and learning materials. Librarians can also be extremely useful as resource personnel when attempting to track down suitable materials or information.

If this venture has the support of the staff, the learning experience can become enjoyable and is likely to perpetuate itself. This then allows the sister to take a less prominent teaching role as each nurse becomes more confident (and professional) in how she uses her newly acquired knowledge.

ASPECTS OF TEACHING

It may be useful now to consider three aspects of teaching that may be applicable to the ward, particularly in relation to student nurses who are undertaking clinical experience. The three aspects are:

- one-to-one teaching;
- teaching a skill;
- assessment.

Obviously the treatment of the above aspects will be, to some extent, superficial as space precludes discussion on underlying theories. Nevertheless, certain points can be raised and techniques described that may prove useful to the busy ward sister who may well have to supervise her staff nurses as they begin to take on the teaching of student nurses in an organized way.

For effective and relevant teaching and learning to occur three conditions should prevail:

- There is something of value to be taught.
- There is someone willing to teach it.
- There is someone willing to learn.

It is perhaps the sister who should satisfy herself that these conditions do, in fact, always hold on the ward.

One-to-one teaching

This method is sometimes referred to as face-to-face teaching and is probably the commonest type of teaching that can occur on the ward. What should be asked, of course, is who is involved in the encounter, as it is often one student teaching another with little supervision from the registered nurse.

One-to-one teaching is potentially a very powerful encounter if the appropriate people are involved and the ward sister can exploit it by linking each student to a staff nurse with the purpose of the staff nurse becoming the student's teacher and mentor. Organizationally this may require the staff nurse and student to have the same or similar shift patterns, particularly at the beginning of the student's clinical experience. If this system is considered by the ward sister she should be satisfied that the staff nurse can assume this responsibility. In the early stages the staff nurse may feel vulnerable and, as she may become an important role model to the student, the student may well begin to reflect some of the staff nurse's characteristics. The staff nurse should also realize that she will be mainly responsible for the student's level of performance by the end of the clinical experience.

Although at the beginning of the teaching/learning encounter the staff nurse will have a high practical input, the aim should be to allow the student to practise the taught skills with a minimum of supervision. Thus the sister should be looking for high dependence giving way to minimum dependence on the part of the student, but this must be the result of increasing identifiable skills and not just time served.

The importance of the way nursing care is organized

The organization of the nursing care on the ward may affect how successful or otherwise this mentor system will be, as under the conventional task-orientated method it is very difficult to apprentice a student to a staff nurse. A patient allocation scheme of some type, with the staff nurse and student forming a nursing team or part of one, is likely to be more conducive to one-to-one teaching.

Familiarity with student training programmes

The sister should ensure that the ward staff are familiar with the student training programmes, so that they have an appreciation of how long students have been in training and, perhaps more importantly, what previous nursing experience they have had. This is particularly important for the staff nurse who has undertaken to act as teacher and mentor to the student.

Working through the objectives

The students allocated to the ward will usually have a list of objectives or statements of experience they require. It is useful if the staff can review with the appropriate clinical teacher or tutor the relevance of these objectives and statements from time to time, as they will underpin the staff nurse's teaching approach to the student.

Monitoring the teaching

The sister should monitor the teaching performance of the staff nurse with a view to giving support and guidance. The staff nurse should not be left to 'muddle on'; rather, a frank exchange of views on how the teaching is progressing can be beneficial to both the sister and the staff nurse. Indeed, in the early stages, both the sister and the staff nurse may be lacking skills and knowledge on certain aspects of teaching, but together they can discuss and experiment and increase their expertise.

Planning the teaching

If the encounters between the staff nurse and the student are to be used to effect the sister may have to discuss with the staff nurse how she is going to plan her teaching. Although the environment of a ward can not be controlled to the same extent as a classroom, this does not mean that any ward learning has to be haphazard or fortuitous.

The staff nurse can be encouraged to teach to objectives. These objectives can be derived from any existing formal objectives and from needs identified by the students themselves. The aims of teaching sessions can thus be pre-specified and shared with the student. This will require the staff nurse to consider just what it is she is trying to convey to the student and what she expects the student to know or do following the teaching encounter. She should write these down and discuss them with the sister as such objectives must fit into the philosophy of the training programme and be appropriate for the stage in training. By doing this, the ward can build up a bank of objectives that each student has to achieve to be deemed to have successfully completed the clinical experience.

Many nurse training programmes actually have the objectives clearly stated and the wards teach to them, but the sister has to satisfy herself that the staff nurse's knowledge is adequate to teach to these objectives.

It should be remembered that such teaching opportunities will occur whilst the staff nurse and student are actively engaged in nursing, but there will be times when the actual teaching may need to take place away from the immediate nursing area. This will require the staff nurse to use her discretion skilfully and her time wisely.

(For those wishing to pursue the idea of objectives there are ample texts available, but for an interesting beginning see Mager, 1962.)

Teaching a skill

There is little doubt that nurse training has been built around skills acquisition; these skills are predominately psychomotor skills, often termed procedures. However, the emphasis is now tending more towards education rather than training and other skills are assuming a higher profile within the curriculum, particularly those described as the interpersonal skills. This is manifest in the move toward patient-orientated care as opposed to procedures-dominated care. (For an interesting account of the differences see Pembrey, 1980.)

Although this change in emphasis is to be encouraged, psychomotor skills still have a legitimate and important role to play in the nursing care of patients. The sister should be satisfied that these skills are being blended with the interpersonal skills into competent nursing practice. In the acquisition of nursing skills the student will be able to observe the staff nurse and then know what her own performance should be like.

When the student is about to be taught a specific psychomotor skill a number of points should be considered and answered in the affirmative:

- Is this an appropriate skill for the stage of training?
- Has the student the appropriate background knowledge to the skill?
- Is the teaching situation typical rather than unusual?
- Is the teacher confident in her own knowledge and ability?
- Is the skill to be taught in accordance with the curriculum?
- Is the correct equipment available to carry out the procedure?

It is useful if the staff nurse can make the patient aware that she is instructing a student in the particular procedure and explains any technical terms she is likely to use. The staff nurse may also have to inform the patient that as the procedure is being taught it may take longer than normal. This is particularly important if the patient is already familiar with the procedure.

A simple rule, often overlooked when teaching nurses procedures, is to allow students to view the performance from as near the operator's position as is possible, e.g. over the operator's shoulder or at least from the same side as the operator. Many students are shown from the opposite side from where the operator stands and this gives the student an entirely different perception of the proceedings.

It is during the teaching of ward procedures that the sister may come into conflict with the methods taught in the school of nursing. However, if the sister is satisfied that the method she advocates is both safe and economical, that it causes the patient no more discomfort or distress than the 'official' method, then she should contact the school of nursing and ask to discuss the issue. Indeed, it could be argued that it should have been the sister and her colleagues who were asked to decide on the most appropriate methods for carrying out ward procedures as they are the practising nurses. If the policy makers are removed from daily nursing contact then conflict in the area of procedures is almost inevitable.

Many authors and researchers (for example, Alexander, 1983) have identified the gap between what is taught in the school of nursing and what is actually practised in clinical areas. This can cause problems particularly for the newly qualified nurse. Kramer (1974) found that this was one of the influences on nurses at this level deciding whether to remain in nursing. The English National Board has made recommendations on this issue, encouraging tutors to follow their students much more into wards and units. Other ways of attempting to minimize the theory–practice discrepancy include the appointment of people with a dual role spanning education and practice. (These are sometimes referred to as a joint appointments or teacher practitioners.)

It is interesting that in fact some health authorities are moving away from the traditional system of procedure manuals to one whereby standards for practice are set. The 'acceptable' nursing activity must then follow certain principles and reach particular standards but degrees of flexibility in method are accepted and indeed, in some circumstances, desirable.

Assessment

Most registered nurses would no doubt claim the ability to identify a 'good nurse' from the experience of observing the nurse as she goes about her job. It is interesting to speculate on exactly what it was a nurse was doing to earn the accolade of 'good nurse'. On what criteria was the judgement based? Would patients and nurse managers agree with the registered nurse's conclusions?

In day-to-day living, assessments are continuously being made about numerous things, e.g. next-door neighbours, television programmes and friends and it is often the displayed behaviour that is being assessed, presumably against certain standards.

An assessment procedure is required when registered nurses have to make competency statements regarding the nursing abilities of student nurses. Thus it is important for the registered nurse to know just what it is the students are expected to achieve during their clinical experience. Ideally this information should be available from the training school as clearly stated objectives but, whether or not this is the case, the registered nurse as an assessor has to be fully familiar with the behaviours to be assessed. This usually implies:

- The assessor understands the behaviour to be assessed.
- The assessor can effectively demonstrate the behaviours.
- The assessor can teach the behaviours to another person.
- The assessor can make an objective assessment of the behaviours.

Assessing against standards

To assess effectively, the registered nurse must have standards against which to measure the behaviour or performance, yet setting those standards can be an area of difficulty. In some clinical areas standards are established by the sister though the ideal would involve all ward staff in agreeing and setting them. Standards may be expressed as the minimum acceptable practice, anything below which is considered unacceptable. Alternatively, they can be stated as ideals, or levels to be achieved, depending on such factors as the experience of those involved in the activity and resources available, but again a minimum level would be implicit.

Standards must be frequently demonstrated and monitored by the sister and all trained staff held personally accountable for the achievement of those standards in their own clinical practice. Where standards are openly generated and form an integral part of the day-to-day work of the ward or unit, the role of the assessor is much clearer.

A problem that concerns standards is that of limited resources, especially if this is used to justify falling or erratic standards. In this situation teaching, learning and assessing become extremely difficult. It is part of the role of the sister in these circumstances to say that resources are such that certain standards can not be reached or maintained, since she is ultimately responsible for the nursing care in the ward or unit.

Achieving good personal standards
The registered nurse's own standards are likely to be satisfactory if she:

- strives to keep her own knowledge base up to date;
- practises her craft and critically analyses her own performance;
- invites constructive criticism from patients and colleagues as appropriate;
- appreciates that basic nursing is a skilful art;
- refuses to trade off standards to save time and resources;
- strives to see both the patient's and the student's point of view.

Priorities and concerns in assessment
The assessor's first consideration is safety. Can the student, after teaching and practice, be left to practise the skill unsupervised, despite the inevitable 'rough edges'? If the assessor is not convinced that the student will be safe then she has a duty to make this clear to the student and to indicate further what exactly is missing from the performance to deem it unsafe. This usually entails further teaching – or opportunities for the student to improve their performance.

To assess effectively the registered nurse should work with the student over a period of time, demonstrating clearly what the student has to become proficient in. This can be followed by supervised practice whereby the registered nurse is closely observing the student's performance and only intervening where necessary. The length of supervised practice that is necessary before formal assessment depends on many factors including:

- the performance of the student;
- the registered nurse's teaching methods;
- the complexity of the skill;
- the danger factor;
- ward and personal standards.

Assessment inevitably carries a responsibility on the part of the assessor and this looms large particularly when a student cannot reach a minimum acceptable standard. The question of failure, a repeat of the experience or even the termination of training, will no doubt be in the assessor's mind from time to time. Nevertheless, the assessor's role is a vital one in highlighting the nurse who is not competent to practice. Some assessors may fear the consequences of failing a student, but they should never be tempted to allow a student through the process in the hope that someone else will stop them. Passing a student who should have failed is a compromise of standards – something that should be unacceptable to any professional nurse.

METHODS TO FACILITATE LEARNING

As has already been indicated learning can occur as a result of many different processes; for example, from experience, by working alongside and observing others, by practising a skill, by one to one teaching, by individual study and by taking part in events such as courses, study days, seminars and discussions. Whilst all of these have a part to play, some are more appropriate in certain situations and to achieve particular learning. However, in general – and especially in continuing education – there has been a move away from the straightforward imparting of knowledge by lectures, and a greater use of groups with feedback and discussion, plus the use of facilitators with a role to encourage the better match between learning opportunities and the needs of individuals.

Further, in view of the fact that teaching time, and places on courses, are limited, there is more emphasis on distance and open learning, and self-instructional methods, though it is suggested that learning by such means is more effective if there is some element of interaction with a tutor or other such sympathetic and knowledgeable person. In addition there are now numerous teaching aids available such as slide/tape presentations and audio-visual material. (A good example is the video 'Anything for Pain?', produced by Kate Seers and Claire Goodman, and available from the North West Thames Regional Health Authority. This not only informs about pain control but is also an innovative and effective way of disseminating the results of research.)

PATIENT EDUCATION

The chapter has concentrated so far on teaching and learning in relation to trained staff and students, but emphasis is also being placed in nursing on patient education and the role of the nurse in this. This is a natural corollary of the move towards individualized patient care where the patient is involved in the planning and implementation of their own care.

If the sister can implement peer group learning amongst her trained staff and use the mentor–apprentice system with student nurses she will have two useful resources within her ward – an improved knowledge base amongst trained staff and a build up of teaching expertise in those staff nurses who have taken on the teaching of a student. This can then be exploited to increase patient education with the sister being the focal point, owing to her unique position in the ward structure and her influence as an expert in the eyes of the patient.

This type of teaching is different in some respects from teaching nurses as one has a potential group of clients whose knowledge and understanding – and motivation to learn – can range widely. Organizing patient education in a meaningful and structured way requires first an examination of how nursing care is organized on the ward. If the approach is one of task allocation and 'finishing the ward' then it may be difficult to implement a patient education programme, whereas if team nursing and patient allocation are used this lends itself more to patient involvement and education.

When developing a patient education programme it is important to consider the contributions of all those whose role is – at least in part – one of health or patient education. This includes the physiotherapist, the occupational therapist, the dietician, the pharmacist, specialist nurses such as stoma care, diabetic and mastectomy nurses as well as medical staff. A collaborative approach, combining the skills and knowledge of all health-care staff, is likely to make the most use of resources, though the co-ordination of the programme can and should come from the sister.

Each member of the nursing team can play a part in the programme, according to her knowledge and interests. For example, if a ward specializes in respiratory disorders, and one of the nurses has a particular interest in asthma, she could be encouraged to draw together material of use with patients suffering from the disorder, discussing it first with others such as her peers and medical staff. Another way of involving nurses in patient education, at the same time as developing the skills of others, is to arrange for a more junior – or less experienced – nurse to observe when a colleague with expertise is 'teaching' a patient about a particular aspect of the patient's care, for example, prior to discharge.

There is now a wealth of material available – either free of charge or relatively inexpensive – to assist in patient and health education. Nurses will often be familiar with information produced by organizations that relate to patients in their care such as the Colostomy Welfare Group, the Ileostomy Association and the British Diabetic Association. A whole range of information is available from the Health Education Authority and the Royal Marsden Hospital has produced a series of helpful booklets on cancer care and therapies.

Special considerations

The question of level of knowledge has to be considered as has the type of language to be used. For example, informing the headmaster of the local grammar school, who is anxious to get back to work, about how he can cope with everyday living following his recent myocardial infarct may require a different approach when compared to an unemployed manual worker with financial and family problems who smokes and drinks heavily.

There is also the fact that most nurses are female and in their early twenties, unlike the majority of patients that they care for. This in itself may introduce difficulties if the nurse is attempting to teach a patient or client who, in terms of background and experience, is very different, and who is often 'old enough to be her parent or even grandparent'! Also, educating patients may involve nurses having to teach patients and relatives techniques and procedures that many nurses have jealously guarded for years as unique to their role. Indeed there is often a greater challenge to nurses in educating their patients than there is in educating their students. If it is to be worthwhile it requires a strong willingness to share knowledge and skills in a warm and appropriate manner. Thus the sister should encourage discussion amongst staff as to the teaching difficulties – and successes – that are being experienced with patients with a view to seeking the most effective approaches.

Rogers (1969) argues that 'the most socially useful learning in the modern world is the learning of the process of learning, a continuing openness to experience and incorporation into oneself of the process of change'. There is a much greater acceptance now that nursing has to change and develop. Therefore learning – and teaching (or the provision of opportunities for learning) – should be inseparable from the nursing activity itself. But this will only be achieved by individual nurses believing that it should be so with the sister, supported by her more senior colleagues and managers, acting as the main catalyst.

REFERENCES AND ADDITIONAL READING

Alexander, M. (1983) *Learning to Nurse: Integrating Theory and Practice.* Churchill Livingstone, Edinburgh.

Farnish, S. (1983) *Ward Sister Preparation: A Survey in Three Districts.* NERU Report 2, Chelsea College, University of London.

Fretwell, J. (1982) *Ward Teaching and Learning.* Royal College of Nursing, London.

Halsbury, Rt. Hon. The Earl. (1974) *Report of the Committee of Inquiry into the Pay and Related Conditions of Service of Nurses and Midwives.* HMSO, London.

Kramer, M. (1974) *Reality Shock: Why Nurses Leave Nursing.* C.V. Mosby, St Louis.

Lathlean, J., Bradley, S. and Smith, G. (1986) *Post-Registration Development Schemes Evaluation.* NERU Report 4, King's College, University of London.

Mager, R.F. (1962) *Preparing Instructional Objectives*, Fearon Publishers, Palo Alto.

Marson, S. (1987) Learning for change – developing the teaching role of the ward sister. *Nurse Education Today*, Vol. 7, pp. 103–8.

Melia, K. (1987) *Learning and Working: The Occupational Socialisation of Nurses.* Tavistock, London.

Nightingale, F. (1882) Nurses, training of, in Richard Quain (ed.) *A Dictionary of Medicine.* Longman's Green, London.

Ogier, M. (1983) The ward sister as a teacher resource person, in B. Davis (ed.) *Research into Nurse Education*, Croom Helm, Kent.

Orton, H. (1983) Ward learning climate and student nurse response, in B. Davis (ed.) *Research into Nurse Education*, Croom Helm, Kent.

Pembrey, S. (1980) *The Ward Sister—Key to Nursing.* Royal College of Nursing, London.

Revans, R.W. (1964) *Standards for Morale: Cause and Effect in Hospitals.* The Nuffield Provincial Hospitals Trust.

Rogers, C. (1969) *Freedom to Learn.* C.E. Merril, Columbus, Ohio.
Rogers, J. (1977) *Adults Learning,* (2nd edn). Open University Press, Milton Keynes.
Vaughan, B. (1980) *The Newly Qualified Staff Nurse: Factors Affecting Transition.* Unpublished MSc thesis, University of Manchester.

8. Industrial Relations
Dee Borley

INTRODUCTION

Ward or departmental managers are unlikely to be involved in complex negotiations on industrial relations issues, but they have a considerable responsibility for promoting and maintaining good relations, and for dealing with problems smoothly and knowledgeably. If their skills and knowledge are inadequate, or if they fail to recognize the importance of good industrial relations, small local issues can easily escalate into bitter and complicated disputes.

Yet it is precisely at ward level that little consideration is given to preparing the ward manager to fulfil these responsibilities. This chapter, while only an introduction to the subject, will discuss potential areas of conflict that may affect the ward manager, examine how local and national bargaining on pay and conditions is organized, and look briefly at the relevant law and sources of advice. At the end of each section a check list will help ward managers assess the level of knowledge and training they need to achieve competence.

INDUSTRIAL RELATIONS AND THE NHS TODAY

The Chairman of Marks & Spencer, when asked his views on industrial relations, is said to have replied 'industrial relations? I don't know anything about *industrial* relations! I only know about *human* relations'.

This story may be apocryphal, but it is a good starting point from which to examine the complex issue of industrial relations as it affects nursing today. Stripped of all the theories, legal issues and complex arguments, industrial relations is all about how *people* get on with each other at work; not just about manager and staff member, but relationships between any individuals and organizations within the NHS.

It is obvious, therefore, that whatever the legal framework and national or local arrangements, individual style and behaviour will, at some stage, influence relationships within an organization. Different personality 'types' are easily recognizable: the autocratic manager, the truculent shop steward, the indecisive person, the person who is easily upset and the one who easily upsets others; each of these will approach a problem from a different perspective and in a different manner, and the outcome in each case will be different.

Smooth industrial relations cannot be ensured, however, simply by paying attention to human relationships – if this were the case, then surely nurses and other health-care workers, who have been trained to relate to others, and to have insight into their needs and behaviours, should have no problems at all! Yet, as is well known, historically nursing has faced serious industrial relations difficulties, and this is still the case today.

In the United Kingdom, much of the industrial relations practice in the National Health Service has been based on the view that managers and staff can identify common goals and can, through joint national and local consultation and negotiation, work towards achieving their joint aims to prevent conflict which could have a disastrous result for the 'consumers' of the service. It has been suggested that the fact that many managers belong to the same trade union as their staff (a situation almost, but not entirely, unique to the NHS) is evidence of the validity of this view. However, as was seen in the 1970s, this model of industrial relations did not serve all situations. Managers are not always sensible, staff are not always reasonable, and pay, conditions of service, and finance for health care are not always ideal. Add to this the factor of individual variation in attitude and behaviour mentioned earlier, and it can be seen that conflict can and does occur.

Today, when even more pressing problems beset the National Health Service, nurses as the largest occupational group within the service face many areas of difficulty. Pay and conditions of service have always been a source of concern, and despite the fact that the system of national pay bargaining was replaced in 1983 by the establishment of a Pay Review Body, dissatisfaction is still felt about both the recommendations of the Body and their implementation by the government of the day.

Since 1974 the NHS has undergone several periods of organizational change, which have affected successive generations of nurse managers, and influenced the way in which they relate to their staff. The most recent of these, the introduction of general management into the NHS (the so called 'Griffiths' reorganization) has resulted in the implementation of many new systems of management and management structures. In some cases this has resulted in clearer accountability and more efficient decision-making; in other cases, however, managers are uncertain of their responsibilities, accountability is blurred, and decision-making difficult.

One result of this succession of changes is that many middle nurse-managers feel baffled, powerless, and unable to give a coherent view of organizational policy to their staff, who struggle with them to maintain a high level of service in the face of increasing pressure – a pressure that is intensified by the growth of the consumerist movement among their patients and clients, demands for greater professional and public accountability, and managerial and professional demands for quality of care to be measured and maintained.

Nurses of all grades in the NHS are becoming aware that the resources, both financial and human, are in many cases inadequate to meet demand, and that improvements in one area have to be made at the expense of another.

Practices that were previously regarded as sacrosanct within nursing are now being questioned by management auditors: the afternoon over-lap of shifts in general hospitals, for example, or the two-shift system in psychiatric hospitals. Shift patterns are undergoing a general re-examination in many areas in the interests of efficiency. Staff residential accommodation, on which many have traditionally relied, is under similar scrutiny, and nurses are faced with the prospect of finding safe, accessible and reasonably priced accommodation outside the hospital – an almost impossible task in many areas of the country. The demand for more efficient use of hospital beds has led to earlier discharge and higher throughput of patients, with a resultant increase in both the work load of the hospital (coping with more highly dependent patients) and the community service (undertaking the continuing care of patients following discharge).

The demand on the community service may be further increased in the future by the proposals to close the large institutions housing mentally ill and mentally handicapped people, and to attempt to improve their quality of life by assisting them to return to the community. The merits of these proposals are currently the subject of active debate, but it is clear that nurses working with these patients feel considerable anxiety about their own personal and professional futures. Not all authorities have felt able to make constructive and sensitive plans for the management of this change, or to discuss these fully with the staff who will be affected.

The community into which the sick, the elderly and the handicapped will return may be ill equipped to cope with them, and unwelcoming; it is also an increasingly unsafe one in which to work. Increasing levels of violence are reported, affecting nurses in accident departments, community nurses and others. Nurses working in inner cities and in isolated rural areas express concern for their own safety, and often feel that their managers do not appreciate their fears.

These areas of concern are mentioned because they illustrate the tremendous potential for dissent which could affect relations at ward or departmental level. It is perhaps unsurprising that many student nurses do not complete their training, that others leave the profession shortly after qualifying as a nurse, and that others, increasingly dissatisfied, are attracted by the benefits of nursing in the independent sector, both in this country and abroad. This sad wastage only increases the difficulty that many NHS authorities are experiencing in recruiting and retaining suitably qualified and experienced staff.

What of those left behind? How do nurses express these concerns, and how can nurse managers of all grades ensure that smooth relationships and efficient services are maintained?

Many senior nurses are now suitably trained in industrial relations and management skills. They have a sound knowledge of the relevant legislation, the systems of bargaining and negotiation, the role of trade unions and their representatives, and the history of industrial relations nationally and within the work place. They also feel, as executors of health authority policy, that they are confident of their position and powers within that policy, and that it is one which is clear, jointly agreed by management and staff, and provides for fair and equal treatment of all.

Representatives of trade unions and professional associations (hereafter referred to as 'staff organizations') also receive comprehensive training in these subjects; it is therefore very important that the ward manager possesses an awareness of these issues, and is provided with training and advice as necessary.

NEGOTIATION AND BARGAINING AT NATIONAL LEVEL

At the inception of the NHS, staff who came within its control had widely differing salaries and conditions of service. A national system for determining these issues was considered necessary for fair treatment of all staff; this was accepted by the government of the day, the managers and the staff organizations concerned.

The system adopted was the Whitley Council system: a General Whitley Council to agree matters relevant to all staff groups, and specific Whitley Councils to determine pay and conditions of service relevant to certain groups and grades of staff. The Nurses and Midwives Whitley Council was one of ten specific councils established.

In 1983, following several years of difficulty in reaching national agreement on nursing salaries, a new system for determining pay was established for nurses and other paramedical staff, the Review Body for Nursing Staff, Midwives, Health Visitors, and Professions Allied to Medicine. The Nurses and Midwives Whitley Council, therefore, is no longer the mechanism for determining salary levels.

Table 8.1 Examples of issues determined by the General Whitley Council

---

Annual leave – general guidelines

Leave for special purposes – compassionate leave, maternity leave, magisterial and other public duties

Expenses – mileage, subsistence, removal, telephone

Redundancy arrangements

Employee relations – facilities for staff organizations, local consultation machinery, disciplinary and disputes procedures

London weighting allowances

Arrangements arising from NHS re-organizations

Both the General and the Nursing and Midwifery Staffs Negotiating Council comprise two teams of people who meet regularly to negotiate or discuss relevant issues: a management side made up of senior health service managers, civil servants, and government representatives, and a staff side drawn from the organizations who represent staff in the NHS. As an example, the current composition of the staff side of the Nursing and Midwifery Staffs Negotiating Council is given in Table 8.3.

Table 8.2   Examples of issues under discussion by the revised Nursing and Midwifery Staffs Negotiating Council

---

Specific arrangements for annual leave
Lodging charges and abatements
'Skill-mix'
Re-grading of senior educationalist posts
Submission of evidence to the Pay Review Body
   (staff side and management side submit separate evidence)

Table 8.3   Composition of the staff side of the Nursing and Midwifery Staffs Negotiating Council

---

Association of Supervisors of Midwives	1
Confederation of Health Service Employees	4
Health Visitors' Association	2
Managerial, Administrative, Technical & Supervisory Association	1
National Association of Local Government Officers	2
National Union of Public Employees	4
Royal College of Midwives	3
Royal College of Nursing of the United Kingdom	8
Scottish Association of Nurse Administrators	1
Scottish Health Visitors' Association	1
Total	27

Both the General and the Nursing and Midwifery Staffs Negotiating Council issue handbooks with full details of the agreements on salaries and conditions of service.

As these are amended following new negotiations and agreements, details are circulated to all employing authorities and staff organizations. An appeal system exists, in order that any agreements that need clarification at local or national level may be dealt with.

Many hospitals in the independent sector employ staff under Whitley Council terms and conditions. The ward managers in the independent sector should familiarize themselves with the terms and conditions under which they and their staff are employed.

The current system of pay determination

Each year the Pay Review Body considers evidence from the Department of Health and Social Security, the service managers, and all interested parties including staff organizations. It considers factors such as comparability with similar groups, unfilled vacancies, and recruitment and retention, and then submits a report to the government of the day. This report may contain recommendations not only on salary levels, but also on other issues; for example the report in 1986 recommended that a comprehensive review be undertaken of the clinical grading structure in nursing, and this is currently under way.

The government may choose whether to accept the report or not, and if it chooses to accept the recommendations will then decide how they will be implemented.

Examples of government arrangements for implementation include whether any award will be paid immediately, or in stages, and to determine how much funding of the pay award will come from central funds, and how much must be found by health authorities from within their own budgets.

It will be seen that nurses might feel dissatisfaction with this system on two counts: firstly, the recommendations of the Body itself, and secondly, the attitude of government to those recommendations. The latter was certainly the case in 1985, when it was decided to pay the award in two stages. Nevertheless, the attitude of many of the major organizations representing nursing to this system of pay determination is one of cautious approval at the time of writing.

Checklist for ward managers

- Do you have, or have you easy access to, the General Whitley Council and Nursing and Midwifery Staffs Negotiating Council Conditions of Service (Whitley Council handbooks)?
- Are these maintained in a serviceable condition, with the amendments contained in advance letters clearly identified and inserted?
- Do you know how national agreements are implemented within your health district?
- Have you read the current report of the Pay Review Body?

NEGOTIATION AT LOCAL LEVEL

The General Whitley Council recommends that, following the system of joint management and staff committees at national level, local joint consultative and negotiating committees should be established. With the introduction of general management into the NHS, many health authorities have such committees at district and unit level. The functions of these committees are discussed in Section 39 of the General Whitley Council Conditions of Service handbook, which recommends that managers should consult staff about any significant decisions that may affect the well-being of employees. It recognizes the benefits of consultation to both managers and employees, and its importance for the smooth working of the service.

The staff side of these committees may be organized in two ways:

- on an occupational basis, with representatives from each broad occupational group employed locally;
- on an organizational basis, with representatives from each of the staff organizations active locally. Staff representatives should be members of recognized staff organizations, i.e. an organization which is represented on a Whitley Council.

The management side of such committees will vary, but should provide for a broad based 'team' of local managers in order that useful discussion can take place. This is perhaps the key to the effective working of local machinery: staff should have a genuine chance to influence decisions and local arrangements, and not merely receive information on matters that have already been decided by management. Failure to pay attention to this can lead to feelings of frustration and suspicion on the part of staff, and result in poor long-term relations between staff and management.

Table 8.4 Examples of issues for local consultation

Disciplinary and grievance procedures
Procedures for investigating complaints
Equal opportunities policies
Introduction of information technology
Changes affecting the workplace and workforce –
    long- and short-term strategic plans and
    administrative re-organizations
Arrangements for statutory holidays

Checklist for ward managers

- Are you aware how your local and district consultative machinery operates?

- Do you know what issues are currently under discussion?
- How would you ensure that your views are represented in local decision-making?
- Do you receive current information on the outcome of discussions from your organizations representative and from your manager?
- Do you have, or have you access to, copies of local policy agreements on issues such as disciplinary and grievance procedures, and do you clearly understand your rights and responsibilities as detailed in these policies?

THE LAW AFFECTING INDUSTRIAL RELATIONS

The ward manager is not expected to be a lawyer, but a knowledge of the principles of the most important pieces of legislation will enable her to fulfil her role with insight, understand the reason for local policies, and ensure that she does not unwittingly treat staff unfairly or illegally.

It is essential, therefore, that she knows where to turn for information and advice, and what organizations exist to offer that advice and to provide guidance notes and publications. The following list may be of assistance.

The Department of Employment

The DoE issues a series of booklets on employment legislation, covering areas such as redundancies, trade union rights, unfair dismissal, contracts of employment, and redundancy arrangements. These are available free from local DoE offices, together with information on industrial tribunal procedure.

Employment advisers, based at key Regional Offices, are available if further or more specific advice is needed.

The Advisory, Conciliation, and Arbitration Service (ACAS)

Established under the 1975 Employment Protection Act, this independent body offers advice to managers, staff, and organizations, and provides a conciliation service in case of disputes. It publishes various Codes of Practice, concerned with, among other issues, disciplinary procedures, the disclosure of information to trade unions for collective bargaining purposes, and representatives' rights to time off to perform their trade union duties.

The Equal Opportunities Commission

Established by the Sex Discrimination Act 1975, this body is concerned with preventing discrimination and promoting equality of opportunity.

The Commission for Racial Equality

The Race Relations Act 1976 established this commission to police the legislation and to provide guidance.

The Health and Safety Commission

The Health and Safety at Work etc. Act 1974 laid down that employers had a duty to provide safe systems of work and to ensure the health, safety and welfare of employees. Each employing authority must have a written statement of policy on these issues and ensure that staff are aware of its provisions.

The act also established the Health and Safety Executive to police the Act, and laid down the rules for inspection of the workplace by its own inspectors.

Health and safety representatives, elected from among members of staff organizations, have the right to inspect, monitor, and report on conditions in the workplace; they may also contact the Inspectorate directly for advice.

The ward managers employing authority

Many employers within the NHS now regard training in industrial relations as essential for managers, and provide their own courses or make use of those run by other organizations. Very few districts, however, extend this training to ward manager level, and yet it is precisely here that unawareness may exist, for example, of the rights and duties of representatives of staff organizations, the importance of avoiding practices that discriminate on grounds of race or sex, and of the ward manager's responsibilities under the Health and Safety at Work Act.

Personnel departments can provide advice on these issues, and guidance as to how new legislation, such as the Data Protection Act, will affect ward managers. Ward managers are advised therefore to make contact with the Personnel Officer responsible for nursing staff, or for their own particular unit, to discuss these issues.

The Hospitals and Health Services Year Book, published annually by the Institute of Health Services Management, gives the addresses of the Bodies mentioned in this section, and a brief description of their function; it also has information on staff and management organizations relevant to the NHS, and is an invaluable reference aid for ward managers.

Check list for ward managers

- Are you familiar with the provisions of the law on the rights and duties of staff organization representatives, and health and safety representatives?
- Does your authority have an equal opportunities policy?
- Does it provide you with the guidance you need to avoid discrimination in recruitment, promotion, and further training of staff?
- Does your employing authority issue written contracts of employment, and statements of the terms and conditions applicable?
- Are you aware of your responsibilities, and those of your staff, relating to health and safety at work?
- Are you involved in formulating and monitoring policies that ensure safe systems of work?
- Does your employing authority provide in-service training and updating, on industrial relations law as it affects managers at ward level?

CONCLUSION

Nurse managers at ward or departmental level have to ensure a high standard of patient care, but can only do so through the staff who work to them.

They must therefore encourage a healthy industrial relations climate within their area, by ensuring that staff are fully informed of issues that may affect their work or their conditions of service, that they have the opportunity to discuss them in an open and constructive manner, and to make their views heard through their staff representatives. It is a mistake to assume that, because staff are 'quiet', industrial relations are calm – the reverse may be the case!

Nurse managers have to ensure that they act in a fair manner towards all their staff, and that they do not, knowingly or unknowingly, contravene any law or national or local agreement. They should feel competent to deal promptly with issues of concern, either by their own intervention or by referring matters to the appropriate person if they feel they are not within their remit.

If they are aware of these issues, and act within local policy, they should also feel secure in the knowledge that they will receive support from their senior nurse manager; indeed that relationship is crucial to the way the ward manager can be helped to take a lively, informed and pro-active approach to industrial relations.

REFERENCES

General reading

Allsop, J. (1984) *Health Policy and the National Health Service*, Longman, London, esp. ch. 3: From Consensus to Discord: An Overview of Government Policies 1940s–1980s.

Bosanquet, N. (ed.) (1979) *Industrial Relations in the NHS: The Search for a System*, King Edward's Hospital Fund for London.

Dimmock, S. (1985) What role for nurses? *Nursing Times*, 20.2.85.

Salvage, J. (1985) *The Politics of Nursing*, Heinemann Nursing, London.

The Preparation of Senior Nurse Managers in the NHS, Kings Fund Centre Project Paper No. 27, April 1981.

Whitley Council/collective bargaining/pay

Gaze, H. (1986) Pay or patients – take your pick, *Health & Social Services Journal*, Vol. 96, 6 February, p. 171. (the Nurses' and Midwives' Pay Review Body)

McCarthy, Lord (1976) *Making Whitley Work: A Review of the Operation of the NHS Whitley Council System*, DHSS, London.

Sargis, N.M. (1985) Collective bargaining: Serving the common good in a crisis, *Nursing Management*, Vol. 16, no. 2, February, pp. 23–7. (an insight from the USA)

Trade-union activities

Bolger, T. (1984) Forty odd pounds for nothing? *Nursing Mirror*, Vol. 158, 7 March, p. 141. (role of stewards in the NHS)

Dimmock, S. (1983) Face to face, *Nursing Times*, Vol. 79, 31 August, pp. 27–9. (time off for trade union activities)

McKay, H. (1978) New industrial relations training, *Nursing Times*, Vol. 74, 2 November, pp. 1813–14.

Disciplinary and grievance procedures

Disputes procedure – success or failure?: An account of practical experience in the use of the NHS disputes procedure, *Hospital and Health Services Review*, Vol. 77, no. 3, March, pp. 71–4.

Fewtrell, C. (1981) Disciplining our procedures, *Hospital & Health Services Review*, Vol. 77, no. 6, June, pp. 163–7 and Vol. 77, no. 7, July/August, pp. 194–7.

Management and industrial relations

Duncan, C. (1984) How far can management influence NHS industrial relations?, *Hospital & Health Services Review*, Vol. 80, no. 6, Nov. pp. 272–6.

Harrison, S. (1979) Analysing how managers react to individual problems, *Health & Social Services Journal*, Vol. 89, 18 May, pp. 602–4.

Whelan, K. (1983) Breaking the silence, *Nursing Times*, Vol. 79, 4 May, pp. 12–14. (distress caused to senior nurses affected by NHS reorganization)

Young, D. (1983) Management – the roadback to trust, *Nursing Mirror*, Vol. 156, 4 May, pp. 33–4. (Staff communication at local level)

Health and safety at work

Finch, J. (1983) Health and safety at work, *Nursing Mirror*, Vol. 156, 25 May, p. 39.

Racial equality

Alonso, R. (1981) Discriminate? Not us! *Nursing Times*, Vol. 81, 27 February, p. 41.

McNaught, A. (1985) Race relations and the general manager, *THS Health Summary*, Vol. 2(S), May, 7.

In a critical condition (1985) (A survey of equal opportunities in employment in London's Health Authorities, London Association of Community Relations Councils, 20 Vauxhall Bridge Road, London SW1V 25B)

Maternity rights

Coussins, J., Durward, L. and Evans, R. (1986) *Maternity Rights at Work*, National Council for Civil Liberties.

Sweet, Corinne (1986) Who pays for pregnancy?, *Spare Rib*, 174, January 1987, pp. 12–17 (a review of the history of maternity benefit and the issues facing working women – useful for those employed outside the NHS)

Case studies

Good relations, *Lampada*, Vol. 3, spring 1985, pp. 30–1. (cases from the RCN Labour Relations and Legal Department)

What would you do? *Nursing Times*, Vol. 79, 20 April 1983, p. 26. (hypothetical disciplinary interviews)

9. Counselling and Staff Support

Glynis Markham

COUNSELLING AND STAFF SUPPORT

This chapter examines the use of experiential learning techniques with groups of ward sisters/charge nurses attending professional development courses and qualified nurses undertaking specialist clinical courses.

The content caters for students from a wide range of health-care settings, spanning all specialties, within hospitals and the community. The majority of these students will have had little previous experience of exploring their skills in this way or of working in interpersonal skills groups.

The aim of these learning opportunities is not to make counsellors of the students but to explore the use of counselling skills and a counselling model in relation to their leadership and management of people. The opportunity to experiment, analyse, practise skills and different techniques in the classroom, without the pressures and stresses of the working environment, is beneficial and thought provoking. The appropriateness of this approach to learning relies on the use of realistic examples of people management problems, in simulated exercises, that not only provide opportunities for practice, but also stimulate discussion and examination of alternative strategies.

Workshops can be planned in a variety of ways, from a number of sessions of two hours duration to short courses lasting for two to three days. However this is undertaken, learning should be planned to ensure that continuity of the subject matter is achieved and that students progress to a clearer understanding of skills, techniques and strategies.

The counselling process

There is considerable confusion about the counselling process, who counsels, what this process is and what it is not. These dilemmas are explored by Hopson (1978) in a paper examining 'a case for demystifying and deprofessionalising counselling' in which he discusses the acquisition of skilled behaviours and the use of these skills by non-specialist workers such as teachers or health-care professionals who frequently have to function in the role of helper.

This title of helper is also favoured by Egan (1982), in his book *The Skilled Helper*, a practical reference work that uses a problem-solving approach to helping and counselling as well as relating theories and models to methods of effective helping. The debate surrounding the appropriateness of a 'purist' counselling role in the routine of nursing is a key issue to be explored in the workshop. Not everyone needs to be, or can be a counsellor but a wide application of the skills employed by counsellors in the management of people, leadership and team building can be helpful to managers in establishing their role. The counselling process and the application of a model of counselling to nursing will be discussed in more detail in this chapter.

WORKSHOPS

Whatever the structure or model favoured by the facilitator, a workshop for students with little experience of group work, self disclosure and the theories of counselling should begin with some basic experiments in communicating. Exercises that demonstrate the skills and pitfalls of communication are a means of ensuring that all students can tune in to the qualities and skills that they already possess, as well as establishing a base line of common understanding of the subject within the group.

These basic exercises can take many forms and are well described in manuals and handbooks specifically designed for gaming (Brandes, 1977; Hewitt, 1981; North, 1981; Munro, 1983). The most common examples of these provide an excellent warm up for the workshop, leading rapidly into discussion of principles and practicalities.

Introduction and warm up

If the workshop is part of a development course the group may have already had the experience of introductions, where each individual has had the opportunity to present themselves to their colleagues. A variation of this, that makes interesting comparison, is the introduction of a partner to the group, following a brief conversation and sharing of some personal history. Discussion of this experience highlights issues of self disclosure, particularly when a partner asks questions or clarifies information. It demonstrates the need to seek approval or check the detail when telling someone else's story and identifies recall and memory issues in relation to listening and responding.

At this point the basic model described by Egan (1982) of

- attending
- listening
- responding

can be introduced as a framework upon which to proceed. The realization that examples of these skills are present and identifiable from this first, simple, conversation exercise reinforces the students' awareness of their own skill and ability to participate effectively in the workshop.

Verbal/non-verbal communication

The use of exercises that demonstrate ways of enhancing or inhibiting good communication, enables students to identify for themselves verbal and non-verbal behaviours that influence our ability to communicate. Examples of these are short conversations, undertaken in pairs, using a variety of seating positions.

Positioning of chairs and partners, back to back identifies the difficulties of conversing with someone who cannot be seen. The problems of when to stop or start talking, or feelings of being a bore, due to lack of eye contact and non-verbal cues are common – as are the adaptation of seating positions and the incidence of distraction from being able to make eye contact with other members of the group.

This exercise can then progress, partners experimenting, with a variety of seating positions, side by side, face to face, at close proximity with knees almost touching, at a distance of 8 ft apart and with one partner sitting on the floor, the other on a chair. The issues of maintaining a comfortable conversation, at the right distance for individual needs, and appropriate to the circumstances, and without distraction are easily explored.

The session can be completed using other exercises to demonstrate the role of verbal and non-verbal behaviours – one partner carries on a conversation where the other partner is instructed to give no verbal or non-verbal response. The feelings of being boring, discomfort and embarrassment are common, the difficulty of maintaining conversation, eye contact and being non-responsive are also experienced. This is followed by a descriptive exercise where one partner describes to the other how to tie a shoe lace, but does so whilst sitting on their hands. The inability to perform this task without demonstrating movements with the feet or head are common. The inability of individuals to follow the description of a practical skill without visual demonstration is frequently seen and has implications when applied to nursing practice where many of the skills taught rely on a visual presentation to assist consolidation of learning.

The final exercise in this session is a simulation, demonstrating a number of verbal and non-verbal behaviours. It is the first opportunity to introduce the role of an observer, in order to feedback performance and to act as a facilitator of discussion. Two students take the role of participants – one or two take the role of observers. Working in threes or fours the participants play the part of acquaintances, one is seeking peace, quiet and tranquillity, the other is determined to initiate a conversation. In short one has to resist interaction, the other persist. The intensity of this exercise highlights many of the behaviours and strategies that we adopt in such situations. The observers have the opportunity to practise their skills in constructive, descriptive feedback of expression, attitude and behaviour.

Attending, listening, responding

The emphasis on the use of the students' attending, listening and respond-ing skills can be readily explored by the use of such exercises. A useful way of consolidating the information and moving the session on to the next phase is to use small discussion groups, of four to five students – their brief would be to identify the skills that enhance good communication and the factors that have an inhibitory effect on communication. Pre-sentation of their discussions on flipchart paper to the whole group allows a comprehensive summary of all aspects of communication to be covered. One of the important issues that will arise from this discussion is the comparison between the ideal climate and environment for good communication to take place in, compared with the realities of the students' workplace.

Once the students have completed this debate, the relationship between their findings and the basic model of listening, attending and responding can be explored, using their practical experiences to illustrate the theoretical models of communication and counselling.

- *Attending*
  using an open, comfortable posture and position;
  maintaining eye contact;
  avoiding distractions or distracting behaviours;
  leaning slightly forward;
  using non-verbal cues such as nodding the head to denote attention and encourage the flow of conversation.
- *Listening*
  taking note of and tuning in to, the tone of voice;
  use of pauses and silences;
  taking note of the use of gesture, posture and expression concentrating on the content of the information being conveyed.
- *Responding*
  using questions to clarify information and understanding of the issues;
  reflecting back information to demonstrate listening and understanding.

This outline provides a structure from which students can examine their own experiences and enhance their understanding of the nature of communication and counselling. However, when viewed against the detail of Egan's work (1982) the simplicity of this structure can be seen in relation to the complex and often confusing view of what counselling is.

An example of this is demonstrated by what Egan (1982) refers to as active listening and McKay Davis and Fanning (1983) refer to as total listening. It can be seen that this concept contains elements of attending and responding, as well as those identified earlier as listening skills.

Total listening

- maintaining eye contact leaning slightly forward;
- reinforcing the speaker by nodding or paraphrasing;

- clarifying by asking questions;
- actively moving away from distractions;
- being committed, even if you are angry or upset, to understanding what was said.

Students who have explored the reference material in search of clear-cut definitions of counselling and its associated skills have often found these inconsistencies frustrating and confusing. The basic communication and counselling skills workshop should clarify the students' understanding and ability to utilize the theories and concepts of counselling, avoiding the pitfalls of a dogmatic approach to the subject.

Values and attitudes

Having identified the basic skills required in maintaining good inter-actions with people the next stage is to explore values, attitudes and qualities of good counsellors. It is a useful warm up to this discussion if students work in buzz groups, drawing from their own experience of people they would choose to discuss problems with, identifying why, and what qualities emerge from their reasons for their choice.

A typical result from this exercise would be as follows:

Qualities of a counsellor

knowledgeable	confidentiality
non-judgemental	good listener
constructive	understanding
unshockable	life experience
respect	honesty
empathy	time
mature	positive
power	objective

This exercise generates material for discussion of how individuals can utilize these qualities and values. For example the skill of making people feel that you have time for their problem when you work in a busy environment. It will also highlight the dilemma that students have with whether sympathy has a place in counselling or when sympathy has to stop and objectivity and empathy should be used. As with all experiential learning techniques there are many permutations and adaptations of this exercise that are dependent both on the direction that the facilitator wishes to take and the ability and experience of the students.

When the students have identified these qualities and discussed values and attitudes, the definition of what counselling is or is not can be explored. This can be done by the students constructing their own definitions, from their workshop experiences. These can then be compared with some of the commonly used definitions of counselling and key elements of the process identified.

Definitions

A process through which one person *helps* another by purposeful conversation in an understanding atmosphere. It seeks to establish a *helping relationship* in which the one counselled can *express* his *thoughts* and *feelings* in such a way as to *clarify* his own situation, come to terms with some new experience, see his difficulty more objectively, and so face his problems with less anxiety and tension. Its basic purpose is to *assist* the individual to *make his own decision* from among the *choices* available to him.

(Standing Conference for the Advancement of Counselling, 1969)

A way of *helping* people to *find and use* their *own resources* for coping with difficult situations.

(Dick Dawes British Association for Counselling, 1979)

People become engaged in counselling when a person, occupying regularly or temporarily the role of counsellor offers or agrees explicitly to offer *time, attention and respect* to another person or persons temporarily in the role of client.

The task of the counsellor is to give the client an opportunity to *explore, discover and clarify* ways of living more resourcefully and toward greater well-being.

(British Association for Counselling, 1980)

These definitions contain key words related to the counselling process that have already been covered by the workshop, some of which will also be present in students' own definitions.

Counselling and health care

The 'purist' definitions of counselling pose some dilemmas for students who work in health-care settings. Macleod Clark (1981) identified the diversity of patient/client communication needs as a continuum ranging from social interaction through to counselling:

- social interaction
- information
- advice
- reassurance
- discussion of diagnosis, treatment and prognosis
- discussion of feelings
- counselling

The skills and abilities required to fulfil these needs are vastly different at each end of the continuum. Hopson (1978) clarifies this by describing a model of helping strategies:

Helping Strategies

Direct action taking action yourself on behalf of the client, practical help
Giving advice making suggestions about the course of action can and possibly should take
Teaching helping someone acquire knowledge and skills that you think they need
Counselling helping someone to explore a problem so that they can decide what to do about it, this is an enabling process.

He develops this model further by stating that the first three strategies assume that the clients' needs are identified, whereas counselling makes no such assumptions, the purpose of counselling being to identify and clarify problems, create a new understanding of the situation. What is so relevant about this helping strategies model is that Hopson's experience is that often the strategies are used in combination for solving any one problem and that the same skills are used, for example active listening, in all strategies. Students find it a clear and easy way of viewing the way in which their skills are utilized in the workplace.

This basic workshop clarifies any misconceptions and confusions and enables all of the group to establish a common knowledge base. It provides experience and practice in the use of techniques that require student participation, self disclosure and analysis of personal style. Once this base line has been established the workshop can progress to sessions that are specifically designed to examine interpersonal skills in relation to leadership and management of people.

SPECIFIC TECHNIQUES – STRUCTURED EXERCISES

There are numerous options available to course planners, depending on the needs of the group and individual group members. Exercises should be flexible enough to allow students to work within their own capabilities and at their own pace. They can also be designed and utilized specifically to explore issues that arise from within the group.

Self awareness

Self-awareness exercises are useful for building confidence and gaining insight into facets of personal style – they also allow individuals to receive some feedback on the way in which others see them.

This kind of feedback can be handled in a variety of ways, in pairs, small groups or whole group activities. For example, working in small groups each individual is identified as an animal. Group members give reasons for their choice, acknowledging the characteristics and qualities that they equate with their choice.

Alternatively, working alone and then with a partner, the individual identifies personal achievements and accomplishments. In pairs they discuss these and identify the individual qualities that arise from these successful activities. The exercise may be extended into considering what inhibits individuals from utilizing their strengths to maximum effect in their daily life (Johnson, 1972).

The opportunity is therefore provided for individuals to have personal feedback, their peers gain practice in giving feedback and in the second exercise partners use their attending, listening and responding skills in a co-counselling situation.

Whilst examining self and self-image it is also useful for individuals to consider the image of the organization in which they work, both in terms of the environment and the people. This engenders some useful discussion on how the climate and culture of the organization, the attitudes, beliefs and behaviours of the people can affect the personal style of the individual.

Personal style and interaction

Individual style and personal awareness lead on to examining interactions between people. The framework used is one introduced by Berne (1964) who identified different communication styles dependent upon from which ego state the individual was operating. The framework consists of three ego states – parent, adult and child – each with specific characteristics:

- *Parent*: the parent ego functions are beliefs, values and attitudes founded on traditions, responsibilities and moral obligations. It has a caring element that is understanding and helpful but if applied in the wrong circumstances can be smothering, increasing obligations and dependence. The controlling element of the parent ego function can be authoritarian, critical and judgemental but used wisely sets limits, defines and protects standards. Students have little difficulty in relating this to nursing and nursing management as they can readily define from which aspect of the parental ego function some of their colleagues operate.
- *Adult:* the adult ego function is thoughtful. It is concerned with facts, logic and realities. It is an unemotional state which gives and receives information, solves problems and makes decisions. The adult ego state mediates between the other two states and is commonly used by people skilled in defusing conflict.
- *Child:* the child ego functions are feelings. In its adapted element the child ego can be polite, obedient, unselfish and conforming – in its free child state the child ego is fun loving, spontaneous, curious, uninhibited and creative but also impatient, selfish and greedy. In addition to this there is an additional state called 'little professor' which is intuitive but manipulative and cunning (Carby, 1976).

This structure can be utilized by the students to examine their interactions. By drawing structural diagrams representing themselves and other individuals, this concept can provide some revealing and amusing observations on interpersonal relationships. The diagram consists of three circles, representing each ego state, the size of the circle proportionate to the frequency that the individual operates from that state (see Figure 9.1 and 9.2). Once the structure has been drawn, students can identify the ways in which communications take place, for example a communication between the critical parent ego state and the free child ego state can be a common source of conflict. Individuals who find

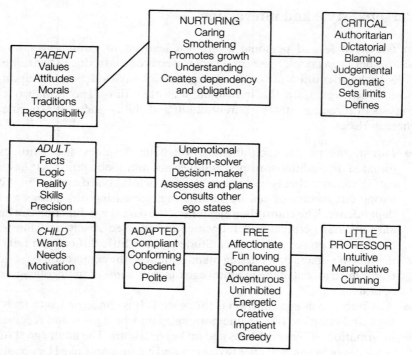

Figure 9.1   Ego state

themselves always operating from an adult ego state with particular people are often doing so to avoid the potential for conflict.

This exercise takes a superficial look at one small aspect of transactional analysis. The potential for using this structure in depth is considerable providing students with a tool for examining both their own, and the behaviour of others, giving them insight into some of their conflicts at work.

Problem-solving processes

Conflicts can also be explored by using Critical Incident techniques (Flanagan, 1954; Clamp, 1980). Working in small groups students are asked to take turns in presenting a work-related problem which they felt had not been satisfactorily resolved. The role of the remaining group members is to use their listening, attending and responding skills to help

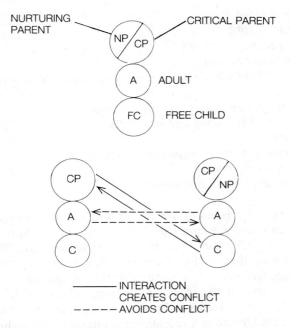

Figure 9.2 Diagrammatic representation of the use of transactional analysis to examine interactions/interpersonal relationships

explore and discuss each problem. The following guidelines are given for the exercise:

● there are no right or wrong answers, only alternatives;
● avoid judgements and identification with the subject;
● be objective, constructive and supportive.

On completion were you

● able to summarize and crystallize the problems?
● identify the emotional from the factual content?

When each problem has been presented and discussed groups are asked to examine and compare their findings with Egan's (1982) three-stage problem management process, before moving on to the next presentation. This process provides an outline for students to discuss and evaluate their progress and effectiveness as helpers.

- *Stage 1:* exploration
  exploring the problem
  focus on specific concerns
- *Stage 2:* new understanding
  seeing self and situation with new understanding and new perspective
  exploring ways of coping more effectively
  identification of strengths and resources
- *Stage 3:* action
  consideration of ways of approaching the situation
  costs and consequences
  plan action, implement and evaluate

By introducing this process at the end of discussion, of the first and each successive problem presentation, it allows students to improve their awareness of their technique by increasing insight into their inherent abilities, reinforcing their skills of analysis and objectivity. Students welcome the opportunity to examine common dilemmas and issues without the pressures of the working situation. This method can be applied to a variety of problems and people-management situations and does not require students to be experienced in interpersonal techniques.

Simulation

More experienced students may wish to 'reconstruct' a situation using group members as participants. The student presenting the problem outlines who the participants are in the simulation and who the other individual/s involved are. The simulation begins with the presenting student talking to an empty chair, which represents the person with whom they have a problem. The conversation revolves around the perceived issue of conflict – when appropriate other students sit in the chair to represent the views of the other person. Other students may stand behind the two individuals acting as supporters, interjecting when appropriate. This exercise represents an interesting, dynamic and participative way of exploring problems, enabling students to identify their feelings, and the feelings of others, in more detail than is normally possible.

Critical Incident techniques provide a methodology for examining issues that may not, in reality, have been satisfactorily resolved. Students may have been unable to discuss the detail of the incident in a critical but constructive framework at work. Classroom discussion encourages objective, informed debate providing the opportunity to consider alternative strategies and approaches in the context of evaluating counselling techniques and skills. Using examples from the work situation ensures that the theories and principles of counselling can be explored in a manner that is applicable to each individual student's professional role.

Stress and anger

Where specific situations are involved, particularly those with an emotionally charged content, such as the management of stress or anger, these can be explored in structured exercises. Working in small groups students can develop their ideas and thinking by identifying the factors that provoke anger/stress and by examining the behaviours and feelings that are elicited in such situations. These findings generate discussion and exploration of strategies for defusing and resolving emotionally charged interactions. This can be followed by the use of specific Critical Incidents and Egan's problem-solving model to provide appropriate subject matter for discussion of skills and techniques suitable for managing such communications.

These incidents can be highlighted by examining and comparing the students' findings with those of Burrows (1984) who identified the following stress factors in the workplace:

- lack of job satisfaction
- unsatisfactory working conditions
- heavy workload
- poor communication
- lack of consultation or participation in decision-making
- poor interpersonal relationships
- 'office politics'

These factors allow students to consider how the environment, culture and interpersonal factors affect the performance of individuals.

Enabling students to gain confidence and practise skills that they can utilize in handling stressful situations is an essential component of any workshop. Burrows' findings are characteristic of the problem factors managers encounter in the workplace. Defining strategies and developing skills that will enable them to foster open, collegiate relationships between team members and reduce the negative effects of these factors can be achieved in a counselling skills workshop. Realistically, stress management may require more time to explore issues in detail – it frequently merits the establishment of a separate workshop to identify individual/team stress factors. Kilty and Bond (1986) have developed a manual of experiential methods to explore stressors and methods of coping with them. The objective being to make stress work for you in a positive manner rather than allowing it to be a destructive force in inhibiting the function of individuals and their working relationships.

Basic counselling skills are clearly essential components in the problem solving, peer support, assertiveness and emotional expression of stress and stress-related problems – using these skills positively to explore and manage the stressors of the workplace will frequently be one of the personal objectives defined by students when considering the value of counselling skills workshops.

Role play

Role play is a natural progression – once students have explored their own examples of problems, the use of specific examples provided by the facilitator can be introduced for simulation. Students who have had little experience of role play, or those who have had previous negative experiences, may be apprehensive but have little difficulty in using triads for simulating role play.

Demonstrations to the whole group are of benefit to generate general discussion but can have an inhibiting effect upon inexperienced students. The facilitator should also be prepared to demonstrate the technique either before or after the students have experimented. Inexperienced students should be encouraged to ignore the desire to giggle and give up their role, being reassured that with practice and persistence these uncomfortable feelings will diminish. Observers are briefed about their observation and feedback role, emphasis is put upon their responsibility to debrief role players with the following instructions:

- Who am I?
- Who I am not?
- Something I like about myself.

The importance of debriefing can be reinforced by the facilitator giving lighthearted examples of 'lurking thoughts', thoughts and feelings that need to be recognized and acknowledged as belonging to the role play and not the player.

It is essential that the facilitator plans scenarios that are flexible enough to be relevant to the student's own role and speciality. This can be done by encouraging students to set their own scenes within the constraints of the brief. For example where an ambivalent student approaches a more senior nurse to discuss the desire to discontinue their course, this could relate easily to basic or post-basic nurse education and it could occur in operating theatres, community care, paediatrics equally as well as an acute or long-stay setting.

The issues and problems explored in the role play are the same, regardless of the setting, and apply to many other common dilemmas, for example nurses with problems in maintaining basic standards of care, nurses with crusading attitudes, nurses with ethical dilemmas, patients or family members handling unfavourable news about prognosis or diagnosis. The wealth of material arising from the conflicts, pressures and problems of the workplace is endless.

If the facilitator is concerned regarding the appropriateness of scenarios to the group's experience this can be remedied by allowing the group to identify the questions and situations they find most difficult to handle, utilizing these as a basis for constructing role-play scripts.

When each role play has been completed the observers give the participants feedback on their performance. The observers' brief is based on a listening, attending and responding skills model. Specific aspects of responding, the use of questions, silence, clarification and reflection can easily be focused on by using these methods.

Additional discussion material can be obtained by using Egan's problem-solving model to examine the progress of the role play in resolution of the issues. If there was not a satisfactory conclusion to the role play, participants should be encouraged to identify the point at which this began to occur and discuss alternative strategies.

Students often voice their doubts about the validity of role play experiences, commenting that it is unreal. The facilitator should explore whether this is because students feel free to express their true feelings in a role play, where those feelings would remain a hidden agenda in reality. Discussion will often reveal students' inhibitions and inability to find ways of expressing these feelings in a non-threatening, conflict free manner at work.

All participants should have the opportunity to function in the role of client, helper and observer. Apart from experimenting with skills and strategies as a helper, or experiencing some of the client's feelings, the observer gains much from close contact viewing of interactions. This experience allows them to be more discriminating, examining alternatives and strategies, selecting and rejecting approaches in relation to personal style. The realization that there are alternatives that work equally well, and that there are no set solutions are some of the benefits derived from observing role play in this way.

Controversial scenarios, such as those with ethical and emotional dilemmas, will provide students with material for discussing judgemental attitudes and feelings generated by individual beliefs and values. This method of experiential learning can be used to explore issues before debating and discussing them in a large group. If this technique is used then some 'ground rules' should be established in relation to disclosure and the use of personal experiences in group discussion.

Video

Video is a valuable aid in encouraging students to develop their observation and discrimination skills. There are many ways of utilizing this facility, some of which will require careful time allocation and planning to achieve a satisfactory and successful outcome.

The use of commercially marketed tapes will provide students with anonymous, non-threatening examples of interviews that they are able to observe and criticize without the anxieties and fears of the consequences and comeback. They provide an opportunity for free, frank group discussion.

If specific issues need to be covered, videos can be made by the facilitators, to role model techniques, or focus on specific subject areas. These can be used in the same manner as commercial material. However, students may experience some inhibitions and sensitivities about constructive criticism directed at the facilitator.

The use of video to give students direct and personal feedback on their performance and style needs careful management. It is difficult to accommodate this kind of experience in short courses – it invariably takes longer than anticipated by the facilitator and a hurried or incomplete experience can negate the value derived by the student.

Role plays between pairs, triads or large groups can be used – students will need to acclimatize themselves to ignoring the presence of the camera before being able to develop their role in the simulation. Viewing can be handled in a variety of ways – this may be dependent on such factors as the experience and capabilities of the group, the group dynamics and the cohesiveness of the intergroup relationships. Ideally the viewing should be shared and discussed as openly as possible to enable the students to practise their diplomatic and descriptive skills as well as learning from the visual replay. Many students will derive considerable benefit from the experience; however, the facilitator should be conscious that some students may get negative feedback both in terms of performance and body image.

THE APPLICATION OF A COUNSELLING MODEL TO NURSING

The use of a helping strategies model of counselling skills has been explored earlier in this chapter – the enabling process of counselling is highly relevant to some of the theoretical discussion concerning nursing models and their application to nursing practice (Orem, 1980); Roy, 1980). If counselling is about promoting the maximum independence and self-determination in the client, enabling them to come to terms with their situation and cope more effectively then there are many aspects of counselling skills that nurses can utilize in providing care and support for patients.

The values and beliefs that nurses have held with regard to the needs of clients and their families have been challenged by the work of nursing theorists. In much the same way the use of counselling skills has challenged the appropriateness of rigid views and judgements in exploring the needs of individuals. There are many parallels between the introduction of nursing models and the use of counselling skills to explore ways of helping clients cope more effectively. The use of such models enables nurses to view their practice with a different perspective, using their skills and knowledge to increase the participation of the client and their family in care, and care decisions.

The use of counselling techniques in the management of personnel, interpersonal and interdisciplinary relationships has numerous possibilities. Students find that the opportunities to examine self and personal style is invaluable in gaining confidence and experience with their own skills, qualities and limitations. Workshops are designed, not just to allow them opportunities to explore their counselling/communication role with clients but to consider its wider application in the handling of staff, group discussions and in particular those issues that generate anxiety, conflict and strong feelings.

The objective of a counselling skills workshop for sister/charge nurses is that whilst practising their skills they should also be able to explore and experiment with ethical and hierarchical issues that arise in their working environment.

Students are encouraged to develop less defensive, non-judgemental attitudes towards situations of conflict simulated in the classroom, to prepare them for their key position as a manager of a clinical area.

Counselling skills can be seen as a tool for nursing practice and management, its techniques are not limited to the exploration of individual client problems but have a wider application in the day-to-day management of people. These skills should be seen as tools to improve and enhance our ability to communicate, enabling nurses to become more effective and sensitive to the priorities of their leadership role.

REFERENCES

Berne, E. (1964) *Games People Play*, Penguin, Harmondsworth.

Brandes, D. and Phillips, H. (1977) *Gamesters Handbook*, Hutchinson, London.

Burrows, G. (1984) *Staff Stress and Burnout–Cancer Nursing in the 80's*, The Cancer Institute/Peter MacCallum Hospital and Royal Melbourne Hospital.

Carby, K. and Thakur, M. (1976) *Transactional Analysis at Work*, IPM Publications, London.

Clamp, C. (1980) Learning through incidents, *Nursing Times*, Vol. 76, no. 40. 2 October.

Egan, G. (1982) *The Skilled Helper*, Brookes/Cole Publishing, Monterey, Calif.

Flanagan, J. (1954) The Critical Incident technique, *Psychological Bulletin*, Vol. 51, pp. 377–8.

Hewitt, F. (1981) Communication skills, *Nursing Times*, Vol. 77, February–October.

Hopson, B. (1978) Counselling – a case for demystifying and deprofessionalising, *Nursing Times*, Vol. 74, no. 2, 12 January.

Johnson, D. (1972) *Reaching Out*, Prentice-Hall, Englewood Cliffs, N.J.

Kilty, J. and Bond, M. (1986) *Practical Methods of Dealing with Stress*, Human Potential Research Project, University of Surrey.

Macleod Clark, J. and Bridge, W. (1981) *Communication in Nursing Care*, HM & M, London.

McKay, M., Davis, M. and Fanning, P. (1983) *The Communication Book*, New Harbinger Publications.

Munro, E., Manthei, R. and Small, J. (1983) *Counselling – a Skills Approach*, Methuen.

North, J. (1981) *Teaching Effective Communication in Nursing*, Rotherham School of Nursing.

Orem, D. (1980) *Nursing: Concepts of Practice*, McGraw-Hill, Maidenhead.

Riehl, J. and Roy, C. (1980) *Conceptual Models for Nursing Practice*, Appleton Century Crofts, New York.

Part Three: Evaluation

10.   Research and Evaluation
Judith Lathlean

INTRODUCTION

This chapter considers two aspects of research – research within a programme and research about a programme. Both of these were pertinent for the Postgraduate Teaching Hospitals Scheme, which sought to enable participants to 'describe and discuss the importance of research and the research process' (Dodwell, 1984) whilst at the same time employing a research strategy to assess the effectiveness of the programme.

RESEARCH WITHIN A PROGRAMME

The exhortation that 'nursing should become a research based profession' – a plea made in the Briggs Report (DHSS, 1972) – is now commonly found in the literature, and reflected in some post-basic and basic education programmes. Yet, as Hunt (1981) asked, 'to what extent has this wish been translated into reality?' Indeed, is research important to nursing and if so, how can 'research mindedness' be developed and research used to improve practice?

The importance of research

Research has been described as 'an attempt to increase available knowledge by the discovery of new facts through systematic scientific enquiry' (Macleod Clark and Hockey, 1979). It is the latter part of this definition which distinguishes it from knowledge gained by other means such as experience or intuition. Yet the dividing line between what does and does not constitute research is not always clear and can depend upon one's view about what is the appropriate foundation for the study of society and nursing in particular.[1] However, it is generally agreed that research should increase understanding of the different aspects of nursing – practice, education and management – either directly or indirectly and in doing so, improve the care given to patients.

Within the context of this general aim, the purpose of nursing research can be varied. For example, although sometimes criticized for 'telling us what is already known', by the use of a systematic approach, research can give credibility as well as testing commonly held assumptions. (An example of the latter is the research on the optimum time for thermometer placement in the taking of oral temperatures: Nichols and Kuchas, 1972, reported this to be nine minutes for women and ten minutes for men at 'normal' room temperatures.)

Research can also be used to evaluate practice and provide a basis for decisions about improvements. If a particular research study is repeated (a process known as replication) this can indicate the applicability of the findings in another setting, or the validity of the initial method. Very often, as well as having the potential to affect practice, research findings can be used in teaching and 'as a springboard for further research'. It is common to find that research studies raise more questions than they answer; thus, they serve to raise the level of awareness and stimulate further study.

The encouragement of research mindedness

If it is agreed that research is important with the potential to enhance practice, it follows that the sister's role in promoting and using research is vital. However, it has been observed that 'in general, nurses as a group . . . are not influenced to any great extent by nursing research' (Hunt, 1984a). Some of the reasons given for this are their lack of knowledge and understanding of research, and their disbelief and inability to apply research findings (Hunt, 1981). Greenwood (1984) took this further and argued that 'findings are perceived as irrelevant to clinical practice . . . because orthodox approaches to nursing research reflect a fundamental misunderstanding concerning the nature of nursing'. It has also been suggested that nursing research cannot be expected to make a difference in practice unless nurses have been encouraged to develop a level of research sophistication which stresses methods rather than results (Wattley and Muller, 1984).

With these points in mind the programme attempted 'to enable [participants] to develop further interest and understanding of research and to appreciate its values and implications in clinical nursing practice' (Dodwell, 1984). It was hoped that by the end of the course the nurse would be able to 'discuss the relationship of research to nursing; describe the research process; critically analyse research findings; describe how research findings can apply to clinical practice; encourage research awareness in other nursing staff and recognise ethical aspects of research involving nurses and patients'.

A variety of methods was used to achieve these aims. Throughout the first series of courses, the programme included sessions on the research process. These stressed the importance of certain strategies in nursing research, for example, particularly those with a strong relationship between research and action and where the complex and changing nature of nursing is recognized and accepted rather than seen as a research 'nuisance' which needs to be controlled. The main aim of these sessions was not to prepare participants for a research role but rather to increase their awareness and 'level of research sophistication'.

Some course members undertook a small-scale project – the emphasis being the utilization of existing research findings and the putting into practice of knowledge and skills gained from the course. However, for a number of reasons, primarily lack of time but sometimes knowledge and motivation, most chose instead to review critically a research project. This appeared to be beneficial and sessions to facilitate research reviews were built into the curriculum.

It is difficult to judge the extent to which the objectives were reached in encouraging research mindedness and research utilization. However, in the evaluation of the programme it was found that participants and their managers identified research as an area in which they benefited.

Utilization of research

If research is to have any impact on practice, it must not be seen as an intrinsically difficult subject which is included in isolation in the curricula of training programmes. It must be viewed as integral to all aspects of the sister's role and patient care. Therefore, this places an onus on contributors to a programme to show just how research enhances knowledge of their subject area, whether it be management of patient care or personnel, or communications or assertiveness skills. This is not to say that there is a wealth of research of relevance to all aspects of nursing; in fact research in nursing is relatively new and in some areas there is a considerable dearth of research information. However, there is research, for example, within the social sciences, and in the study of organizations which can be useful for nursing though there has been a tendency for nursing to be somewhat insular in this respect.[2]

Another way of increasing research awareness and utilization is for the hospital itself to have a system which facilitates its use in practice. The Royal Marsden Hospital has produced a *Manual of Clinical Nursing Procedures* which is 'research based, by using research findings wherever possible to determine policies and procedures' (Hunt, 1984b). It does however point out that unfortunately 'in many areas there is little or no valid and reliable research'. Groups of nurses come together to discuss policies and procedures and thus this has the effect of encouraging them to focus upon, and share knowledge about research.

It probably will be quite sometime before nursing does become a research-based profession; the signs are however that with an increased attention to its importance, and a greater exposure of individuals and groups to research which is relevant to practice, this ideal is achievable.

RESEARCH ABOUT A PROGRAMME

There is an increasing recognition that evaluation should form an important part of all major innovation and change in social settings. This move towards the incorporation of evaluation into new development has been particularly noted in recent years in the field of education but is also gaining momentum in health care generally and in nursing specifically.

To this end, the author worked collaboratively with the project director to devise and implement ways of evaluating the training programme for sisters. The system was piloted, and in part modified, with the results from each stage being used to develop and improve the programme over a period of several courses. Some of the outcomes of this process are highlighted and discussed, and the methods used are critically examined in the hope that they may be of use to others interested in monitoring their own educational innovations.

Issues in evaluation

It is useful first of all to review some key features in order to put the approach chosen for the evaluation into context.

Changing emphasis in evaluation

Views about the nature and function of evaluation in education and training have changed greatly since the 1960s when the purpose was typified as providing 'objective, systematic and comparative evidence on the degree to which the programme achieved its intended objectives' (Hyman, Wright and Hopkins, 1962). More recently, evaluation has been construed more broadly as 'any intervention aimed at providing feedback about the processes and nature of human development, the organisational systems and programmes intended to facilitate it, and the wider organisational context' (Easterby-Smith, 1981).[3]

In essence, the emphasis has moved from attempts to measure externally the effectiveness of the programme alone towards a realization that what is happening – and why and how it is happening – are as important considerations as outcomes. Also, it is insufficient to concentrate only on the inputs and outcomes of the training; of equal importance is the context within which the training takes place and the processes of learning. These include structural considerations such as the location of the training and the factors appearing to stimulate or inhibit learning, and cultural, such as the values inherent in the programme.

Implicit in this is the acknowledgment of 'the intentionality of human action, the importance of subjective opinions and perspectives, and the possibilities and implications of multiple realities within an institution' (Parsons, 1976). Thus it is insufficient, and inappropriate to rely on the 'objective' data of the external researcher. Rather it is crucial to examine a situation from a number of perspectives, including the experiences of the participants.

There is an increasing use of forms of evaluation whereby the results of the evaluation are used to help develop the programme as it proceeds. Indeed, the importance of evaluation in providing feedback when planning and implementing change in many settings, not just educational programmes, is stressed by several writers on the subject including those in Hollingworth (1985). Above all the plea from evaluators and policy makers alike is for evaluation that is useful (Patton, 1982), which can be achieved in part by using the results to influence further development, and also by ensuring that the aims and methods used give rise to data which are policy relevant (Patton, 1978).

Feedback and development

A distinction is sometimes drawn between 'summative' and 'formative' evaluation (Scriven, 1967). To the summative evaluator, the outcome of the programme is the focus of his work, and he seeks to answer the question, 'Did the programme work?' On the other hand, the formative evaluator works through the programme to gather information aimed at improving its operation and provides regular feedback on the planning and implementation of the programme. Such an approach seems to have merit when one of the purposes of evaluating is to improve practice.

The tenets of formative evaluation are in line with an action research approach but the latter goes further in advocating not only feedback to influence decision-making about changes to the programme, but also the importance of a collaborative relationship between evaluator and practitioners and an involvement of the researcher(s) in the policy-making process. There are many different action research models but most exhibit these aforementioned features.

Action research has been particularly advocated for use in situations of change since it can incorporate elements of evaluation and developmental consultancy. However, it does require a considerable investment of time and, where an external independent researcher is involved, a high degree of continuous collaboration between researcher and practitioners. Where this is not feasible (as was the case with the evaluation of the Postgraduate Teaching Hospitals Programme since there were no additional resources for external evaluation) an alternative can be employed which has many of the same advantages. This is the form of action research used sometimes in education (see for example, Elliott, 1981), whereby the practitioner acts (in part) as researcher. This was found to be particularly relevant in relation to the evaluation of this programme: the project director worked collaboratively with the researcher in the development and modification of the evaluation methods but herself undertook much of the data collection.

The responsibility for evaluation

Consideration of who undertakes the evaluation raises the issue of the responsibility of those creating change. Nisbet (1975) identified three main requirements for successful innovation – involvement, support and evaluation. He argued that in the long run innovators will be called to account for their plans and actions and suggested that this should be planned for with an initial incorporation of recording systems into the action. And there is certainly evidence of collaborative research and evaluation being undertaken within nursing education whereby researchers and practitioners work together to assess the merit of an innovation and to share in its development. For example, the author has been involved in two projects whereby innovatory training schemes have been set up with integral evaluation performed jointly by external researchers and staff participating in the ventures (see Lathlean and Farnish, 1984 and Lathlean, Smith and Bradley, 1986).

It is likely that with the current concerns of ensuring value for money, ascertaining the most efficient and effective use of scarce resources, alongside the desire to improve standards, evaluation will be an essential feature of most new developments.

The purpose of evaluation

The aim of much contemporary evaluation is to illuminate and describe the issues involved in an innovation rather than to attempt a precise measurement of outcomes. Similarly, the purpose of the evaluation of this programme was to ascertain the benefits deriving from the training programme and to explore the features of the scheme that appeared to promote development. It was also envisaged that the information gained would assist in the modification and improvement of the scheme.

Inevitably, where resources for evaluation are limited, as here, the focus is on particular aspects of the innovation. In this instance, the initial orientation of the evaluation was the participants' (sisters') perceptions of the course and the extent of their knowledge and skills in various aspects of the sister's role at the end of the course. This was modified during the programme to include a greater emphasis on the needs of course members and the extent of their development during the programme. Although the contextual aspects of the scheme and the viability and effectiveness of the particular features of the programme were considered important, it was regrettably not found possible to study these in any depth.

The evaluation in practice

In the belief that evaluation should be 'active – reactive – adaptive' (Patton, 1978) the methods used were modified over time but many of the principles described above were adhered to throughout the evaluation of the programme. The process involved elements of evaluation and assessment, and included data collected by – and from – many different people such as the project director, facilitators, managers and course members, with guidance from initially one and subsequently two research advisers.

The project director played a key role in managing the evaluation overall including the two main aspects of:

- the evaluation of the course by course members;
- the assessment of course members' performance by themselves and others.

The information gained from these was essentially complementary in helping to build a picture of the success – or otherwise – of the programme but each had a particular purpose.

Course members' perceptions of the course

To assess how well the course was meeting the needs of the course members, participants completed evaluation questionnaires during each week's module. Members reflected on the adequacy of prior information received, and were asked to identify those sessions which were most – and least – beneficial to them with comments on presentation and the main points learnt. This process was reinforced by the structured opportunity to review every module on its final day. This served the dual purpose of gaining feedback about the more 'formal' part of the course and involving participants in a dialogue which could often lead to modifications to the programme.

Assessment and performance review of course members

The dangers of attributing a change in, for example, a person's behaviour solely to the experience of a course is well documented in the evaluation literature (see Easterby-Smith, 1981). However, even if the causal relationship between course and behaviour (i.e. input and output) is elusive it is possible to examine in detail aspects of this by looking at such factors as the needs of individuals, the objectives of the course and the level of achievement of individuals in relation to these aims.

The evaluation set out with this aim, utilizing the experience of a previous evaluation of a training scheme for sisters (Lathlean and Farnish, 1984). Two forms were devised, one specifically for completion by facilitators in relation to interviews conducted with course members and the other designed to match course objectives with individual performance.

The *facilitator's interview form* allowed for the recording of the main points of three interviews held between facilitators (specially designated personnel – education staff and managers – in each of the participating hospitals) and course members. The purpose of the interviews was to ascertain the needs of individuals and to encourage the discussion of progress and problems. The benefits of these discussions lay more in the opportunity they provided for individual support and review rather than the information gained for overall evaluative purposes. Understandably the recording was variable and secondary to the main aim. Nevertheless, they have proved to be a source of useful feedback for the project director.

The *assessment and review form* attempted to relate the course to the performance of individuals by matching the course objectives – which were clearly specified at the outset – against the standard reached by participants. In this way, it was hoped to gain some 'measure' of achievement, and an idea of further learning needs. The initial version of this form was completed at the end of the sixth month of the course by the facilitator and/or the manager and discussed with the course member, with the 'assessor' being required to judge, and justify their judgement about the standard reached in a large number of aspects of the sister's role. Figure 10.1 shows a sample page of this form.

Such a system was found to work well in another ward sister training scheme (Calcott, 1982) but a few problems were experienced in its use in this instance. For example, the form was felt to be long and detailed and therefore time consuming to complete. Also, it provided little indication of changes occurring in performance during the course, added to which the main focus was the standards of a particular facilitator or manager.

As a result of reviewing its use, the form was reduced in length, simplified and oriented towards change and development over time as well as the level of performance of the course member. And, in addition, the focus was shifted more towards initial self-assessment by course members compared later with the facilitator's manager's views.

The revised system has two forms, one to be filled in prior to the course member starting the course and the other for completion at the end. The items – reduced from 67 in the original version to 36 in the revised – are identical for both forms. However, the questions asked are different. In the pre-course form course members are asked to consider the extent to which they need to learn about the various elements of their role – a great deal, some aspects – or are they already sufficiently skilled or knowledgeable? Their own assessment is then discussed with their immediate superior or the facilitator and any discrepancies noted. In the post-course form, individuals judge the extent to which they have learnt or improved – a great deal, to some extent – or has there been no change or even a deterioration? Again the individual's assessment is discussed with the facilitator or manager. Figure 10.2 illustrates this with a sample page from the two forms.

The information collected by these methods is confidential and shared only with the project director and research adviser. Since the main

Clinical nursing management	Tick column where applicable					
	Outstanding	Good	Satisfactory	Average	Unsatisfactory	N/A
● Discusses the philosophy of nursing and identifies principles of clinical nursing management.						
● Outlines a nursing model upon which he/she bases his/her practice and is able to justify his/her decision.						
Conducts a satisfactory nursing assessment.						
Identifies patients' problems and uses a problem-solving approach in patient care.						
Plans realistic care plan.						
Ensures nursing care is carried out.						
Recognizes and develops tools for evaluating such care.						
Participates in maintaining accurate written records.						
Is aware of the ethical and legal implications in the treatment and care of patients.						
Behaves professionally.						

Could facilitators and course members please use different coloured inks when ticking, and state their colours for ease of identification.

Figure 10.1   Sample page from an assessment form: original system.

purpose is to aid an evaluation of the programme, completed forms are not included in the sister's personal file nor do they supersede the normal appraisal and assessment systems in the hospitals (see Chapter 5).

A further aspect of the assessment of course members was undertaken through the written work forming part of the course, in particular essays on the role of the sister, preparation of an audio-visual aid, case or care studies, a research review or a small research project. Various of these assignments were submitted during the course, giving an indication of the learning that was taking place and developments occurring in writing skills. This provides a somewhat tangential, but valuable, method of estimating the effectiveness of the course in terms of certain knowledge and skills gained.

The results of evaluation

Although the information that could be used to judge the effectiveness of the programme came from a variety of sources, the main ones were the evaluation questionnaires completed by course members, the review sessions forming part of the course, the interviews held between participants and facilitators, and the communication between managers and project director. And such feedback proved to be very worthwhile, particularly in indicating the extent of match between individual needs and the course and in suggesting constructive ideas for improvements to the programme.

Participants' perceptions of the programme

From the evaluation questionnaires, the answers to questions about the most and least beneficial subjects were interesting. In an analysis of responses gained from the first series of courses, there was considerable common ground in the subjects chosen as most beneficial with six subjects being listed by over half of all respondents. These were communications, research, counselling, assertiveness training, legal aspects and discipline and grievance.[4] This concurs with the findings of Lathlean and Farnish (1984), in their evaluation of a ward sister training scheme, where the three most frequently mentioned topics of most benefit were research, counselling and communications. Further, Farnish (1983) noted that a very high proportion of her sample of sisters (81 per cent of a total of 166) had felt inadequately prepared on appointment to tackle 'issues concerned with industrial relations' and over half to 'counsel members of the ward team'.

Assessment form 1

Clinical, ward and personnel management

	Please tick column when applicable			
	Needs to learn a great deal	Needs to learn some aspects	Is already sufficiently knowledgeable/skilled	N/A	Comments

- Ability to discuss the principles of clinical nursing management.
- Ability to outline and justify a nursing model upon which my practice is based.
- Awareness of the ethical and legal implications in the treatment and care of patients.
- Ability to communicate effectively with:
   patients
   relatives
   staff
- Knowledge and ability to apply effective leadership skills.

Assessment form 2

Clinical, ward and personnel management	Please tick column when applicable				
	Improved/learnt a great deal	Improved/learnt to some extent	No change	Deteriorated to some extent	Comments
● Ability to discuss the principles of clinical nursing management.					
● Ability to outline and justify a nursing model upon which my practice is based.					
● Awareness of the ethical and legal implications in the treatment and care of patients.					
● Ability to communicate effectively with: patients relatives staff					
● Knowledge and ability to apply effective leadership skills.					

Figure 10.2 Samples pages from pre- and end-course assessment forms: revised system.

The spread of subjects considered to be least beneficial was greater, but those referred to most frequently included information about the statutory bodies and multidisciplinary teams, interpersonal skills and the practical responsibilities of the sister. In addition, some subjects were mentioned as both least and most beneficial by different members in the same group. They included research (again comparable with the findings of Lathlean and Farnish, 1984), computers, the nursing process and bereavement. It appeared that there were many reasons for these divergences of opinion including personal preferences, previous knowledge and experience of the subject, views held as to what is important for the role and actual differences in the roles and needs of individual course members. The method used was also an influence in determining the degree to which participants felt they learnt about the subject with experiential methods and discussion taking preference over didactic lecture approaches. (This finding is borne out in many studies of the most appropriate ways for adults to learn.)

Benefits of the programme

The majority of participants in the first series of courses felt positive about the experience of the course and many were encouraged when returning to their hospital 'to look at ways of improving patient care'. The following comment of a course member summarizes those of many others: 'I feel that I am beginning to be better equipped to fulfil my role as sister.' For some it was indeed a revelation as to what the role actually entailed, the course proving to be 'a real eye-opener . . . particularly into the various aspects of management.'

The specific features of the course were commented upon including the importance of the opportunity to be away from the pressures of the ward or unit, and the chance to be able to 'stand back and view [your] own faults' in an environment where revealing weaknesses was acceptable and 'safe'. The discussion of principles as well as practical detail was valued, and some contrasted the approach used in the programme with less favourable experiences of other management courses which tend to 'bear little relation to reality'.

The issue was raised of whether the course was equally relevant for specialty as for general sisters. In the main participants could appreciate the common aspects of sisters' roles whatever the clinical setting. Even those who had been unconvinced initially that the course would be 'suitable for them' (such as sisters from paediatrics, theatres and psychiatry) conceded that 'even if you don't have to deal with relatives, for example, you're dealing with people and many of the same principles of interpersonal skills are the same'. On the other hand some felt better equipped to start with than their peers, for example, sisters in psychiatry sometimes had greater previous experience of counselling and related skills and considered the level of course input to be inappropriate for them.

Greater motivation and interest to pursue reading and further study on subjects was referred to by many participants which could lead to a desire to 'institute new ideas in the clinical situation and extend [this] enthusiasm to others'. It was possible to identify a number of changes stimulated by the course; for example, the introduction of structured teaching sessions, regular ward meetings and staff support groups, and the starting of a small research project. Yet, in some instances, course members expressed frustration at their inability to put into action some of what they learnt because of organizational constraints, such as the blocking of change by managers, the shortage of resources and manpower, the lack of personal authority to achieve such a change and the attitudes of other people important in ensuring the success of the innovation. It is not uncommon to find this difficulty but it sometimes points to the need to look closely at strategies for facilitating change (the translation of theory into practice), in addition to concentrating on the learning input and experience.

Most of the feedback from individuals was positive, ranging from comments such as: 'I will remember these four months as being the most enjoyable and thought provoking of any nursing course I have undertaken' to those which were still positive but less euphoric, such as: 'Management in broad terms does not excite much enthusiasm but I can honestly say that there has been no subject which hasn't proved interesting.' Nevertheless, many had difficulty in assessing the actual effects of the course on the ward work. The revised assessment system has not been used for long enough to gain sufficient feedback but the perceptions of managers are illuminative in this respect.

Managers' reactions

Managers in each of the participating hospitals have been asked to comment on developments they have noticed in course members attending from their hospital. Although there are problems in trying to compare participants' behaviour before and after the course, particularly as some were newly appointed sisters on commencement and therefore previously occupied a different role, it was possible for managers to identify a number of important changes in their nurses.

A common theme throughout their replies was that of increased knowledge and skills amongst participants, both the relatively inexperienced and experienced. A greater awareness of legal and ethical issues, improved communication skills and a better approach to the management of staff were specifically mentioned in respect of several course members. Accompanying these developments was a general increase in confidence for virtually all participants and in addition, some course members who appeared to have certain problems, such as an inability to delegate or a reluctance to teach, were showing signs of improvement. These positive signs were not always recognized by the course members themselves, but in turn, some of the changes that they saw in themselves were not always apparent to their managers.

Course members often referred to their increased understanding of the sister role and this was confirmed by the managers who detected a development of greater insight in many of their sisters. Also there was evidence of an awareness of the areas of responsibility of sisters which included the ability to identify and diffuse problems at an early stage and the need to evaluate practice.

Third, changes in the attitudes of the sisters were noted, for example, higher levels of motivation and enthusiasm, an increased tendency towards creative thinking, and the acceptance of the need for change and development on the ward.

Managers did point out, however, that there was still need for further help for several of the nurses, for example, in terms of the support needed in handling difficult management situations and in developing their ward teaching.

Finally, several of the managers considered that the increase in the number of applicants for the courses after the first few courses was an indication of its perceived value.

The worth of evaluation

Evaluation as an integral aspect of an innovation is of value not only in assessing the effectiveness of the innovation but also in providing a mechanism for the feedback of results and a basis for further policy decisions. Evaluation procedures must be 'active – reactive – adaptive' (Patton, 1978) to match the nature of change in nursing particularly at a time of maximum uncertainty about a whole range of factors with the potential to affect nursing practice, management and education. Certainly the evaluation of this programme has both provided an indication of its successful and less successful features, and has contributed to its development.

Although there are some advantages to a totally independent evaluation (as was suggested at the outset in the planning stages of the scheme), there are also considerable benefits from a collaborative venture, where those responsible for the innovation are in effect the evaluators but with advice, support and input from external sources such as persons with special skills in evaluation research.

It is too early to be sure whether the revised system for evaluation will prove to be the best way of evaluating the programme, but the initial reaction seems to be that the system is more meaningful and manageable and therefore more likely to be producing useful information. It is the kind of system that could fairly simply be built into different training programmes (for example, a similar approach has been used in the evaluation of schemes for the professional development of newly registered nurses, Lathlean, Smith and Bradley, 1986). Also, the system could be adapted for use in other settings, for example the community, by following the same principles but related to the relevant role.

Such a system appears to have various benefits over and above the assessment of the performance of individuals. For example, it encourages nurses to examine critically their roles and brings together individuals and their managers to discuss performance and progress. This can provide a useful source of support particularly when other studies have shown that one of the most important aspects of schemes for the development of trained staff is the provision of support in the implementation of their roles (see for example, Runciman, 1983 and Pembrey, 1980).

Many writers on educational evaluation have described the activity as stopping short of making judgements of worth as in the following definition: 'Curriculum evaluation is the collection and provision of evidence on the basis of which decisions can be taken about the feasibility, effectiveness and educational value of the curricula' (Cooper, 1976). However, in this instance it was considered more appropriate to follow the maxim of Scriven (1967) and White (1971) and use the evaluation, at least in part, unashamedly to 'judge the worth of [the] programme'.

CONCLUSION

Research occupies an important role in nursing. In this context it spans both the attempt to increase the research awareness of the programme participants and the encouragement to use research findings in practice and the evaluation of the programme. Nursing has some way to go before it becomes a research-based profession, since there is evidence to suggest that nurses lack the knowledge, ability and motivation to apply research. However, strategies to facilitate this can be built into training programmes.

Evaluation of programmes is an increasingly common feature, both to judge the effectiveness and to assist in their improvement. Methods can be employed which ascertain individuals' perceptions of the programme and identify aspects of their roles in which development is both needed and appears to occur.

NOTES

1. For the interested reader further explanation can be found in Lathlean, Smith and Bradley (1986) pp. 13–15.
2. A good example of the appropriate use of non-nursing research and literature is found in Pembrey's (1980) study of the ward sister's role. This study was firmly grounded in organizational theory.
3. The relevance to nursing of these changing views about approaches to evaluation has been summarized by Lathlean and Farnish (1984).
4. This finding was at least partially influential in the choice of chapters for this book.

REFERENCES

Calcott, R. (1982) Evaluation, assessment and appraisal, in H.O. Allen (ed.) *The Ward Sister: Role and Preparation*, Baillière Tindall, Eastbourne.

Cooper, K. (1976) Curriculum evaluation: Definitions and boundaries, in D. Tawney (ed.) *Curriculum Evaluation Today: Trends and Implications*, Schools Council Research Studies, Macmillan, London.

Department of Health and Social Security (1972) *Report of the Committee on Nursing* (Brigg's Report), HMSO, London.

Dodwell, M. (1984) *London Postgraduate Teaching Hospitals Ward Sister's Training Project: The Report* – May 1983–December 1985, The Royal Marsden Hospital, London.

Easterby-Smith, M. (1981) The evaluation of management education and development: An overview, *Personnel Review*, Vol. 10, no. 2, pp. 28–36.

Elliott, J. (1981) *Action Research: A Framework for Self-Evaluation in Schools* Schools Council Programme 2: *TIQL Project,* Working Paper no. 1.

Farnish, S. (1983) *Ward Sister Preparation: A Survey in Three Districts,* NERU Report no. 2, Nursing Education Research Unit, Chelsea College, University of London.

Greenwood, J. (1984) Nursing research: a position paper, *Journal of Advanced Nursing,* Vol. 9, pp. 77–82.

Hollingworth, S. (1985) *Preparation for Change,* Royal College of Nursing, London.

Hunt, J. (1981) Indicators for nursing practice: The use of research findings, *Journal of Advanced Nursing,* Vol. 6, pp. 189–94.

Hunt, J. (1984a) *Nursing Research: Does It Make a Difference?* Unpublished Paper, International Conference of Nursing Research, Imperial College, London, April.

Hunt, J. (1984b) From the Introduction of Pritchard, A.P. and Walker, V.A. (eds.) *The Royal Marsden Hospital: Manual of Clinical Nursing Policies and Procedures,* Harper & Row, London.

Hyman, H., Wright, C.R. and Hopkins, T.K. (1962) *Applications of Methods of Evaluation,* University of California Press, Berkeley.

Lathlean, J. and Farnish, S. (1984) *Ward Sister Training Project,* NERU Report no. 3, Nursing Education Research Unit, Chelsea College, University of London.

Lathlean, J., Smith, G. and Bradley, S. (1986) *Post-Registration Development Schemes Evaluation,* NERU Report no. 4, Nursing Education Research Unit, King's College, University of London.

Macleod Clark, J. and Hockey, L. (1979) *Research for Nursing: A Guide for the Enquiring Nurse,* HM & M, London.

Nichols, G.A. and Kuchas, D.H. (1972) Taking adult temperatures: Oral measurements, *American Journal of Nursing,* Vol. 72, pp. 1091–2.

Nisbet, J.D. (1975) in S. Hollingworth (1985), op.cit.

Parsons, C. (1976) The new evaluation: A cautionary note, *Curriculum Studies,* Vol. 8(2), pp. 125–38.

Patton, M. (1975) *Alternative Evaluation Research Paradigms,* University of North Dakota Press.

Patton, M. (1978) *Utilization-Focused Evaluation,* Sage, Beverly Hills, California.

Patton, M. (1982) *Practical Evaluation,* Sage, Beverly Hills, California.

Pembrey, S.E.M. (1980) *The Ward Sister: Key to Nursing,* Royal College of Nursing; London.

Runciman, P. (1983) *Ward Sister at Work,* Churchill Livingstone, Edinburgh.

Scriven, M. (1967) The methodology of evaluation, in R. Taylor *et al., Perspectives on Curriculum Evaluation,* AERA, Rand McNally, Chicago.

Wattley, L.A. and Muller, D.J. (1984) *Teaching Research: A Practical Approach,* unpublished paper, International Conference of Nursing Research, Imperial College, London, April.

White, J.P. (1971) The concept of curriculum evaluation, *Journal of Curriculum Studies,* Vol. 3 (2), pp. 101–12.

Further Reading

CONTINUING EDUCATION/PROFESSIONAL DEVELOPMENT

Agyris, C. and Schon, D.A. (1980) *Theory in Practice: Increasing Professional Effectiveness*, Jossey-Bass Publishers, London.

Cooper, S.S. (1980) *Self Directed Learning in Nursing*, Nursing Resources, Wakefield, Massachusetts.

Cooper, S.S. (1983) *The Practice of Continuing Education in Nursing*, Aspen System Corp., Maryland.

Cooper, S.S. and Neal, M.C. (1980) *Perspectives on Continuing Education in Nursing*, Nurseco, Inc., Pacific Palisades, CA.

Houle, C.O. (1980) *Continuing Learning in the Professions*, Jossey-Bass Publishers, London.

Smyth, J. (1985) Developing staff development, *Senior Nurse*, Vol. 2, no. 1, pp.14–15.

Tobin, H., Wise, P. and Hull, P. (1979) *The Process of Staff Development: Components for Change* (2nd edn), C V Mosby, St Louis.

Working Party on Continuing Professional Education and Professional Development for Nurses, Midwives and Health Visitors (1981) *Continuing Education for the Nursing Profession in Scotland (The Auld Report)*, SHHD, Edinburgh.

TRAINING AND DEVELOPMENT FOR SISTERS

Allen, H.O. (ed.) (1982) *The Ward Sister: Role and Preparation*, Baillière Tindall, London.

Farnish, S. (1985) How are sisters prepared? *Nursing Times, Occasional Paper*, Vol. 84. no. 4, pp. 47–50.

Lathlean, J. (1986) Education and training for sisters, *Nurse Education Today*, Vol. 6, pp. 158–65.

Lathlean, J. (ed.) *Research in Action: Developing the Role of the Ward Sister*, King's Fund, London.
Pembrey, S. and FitzGerald, M. (1987) Developing the potential of sisters, *Nursing Times*, Vol. 83, no. 12, p. 27.

ASPECTS OF THE SISTER ROLE

King, P. and Dalton, P. (1987) Researching the ward sister role, *Health Care Management*, Vol. 2, no. 3, pp. 27–31.
Marson, S. (1982) Ward sister – teacher or facilitator? An investigation into the behavioural characteristics of effective ward teachers, *Journal of Advanced Nursing*, Vol. 7, pp. 347–57.
Matthews, A. (1982) *In Charge of the Ward,* Blackwell Scientific, Oxford.
Ogier, M. (1986) An ideal sister – seven years on, *Nursing Times, Occasional Paper*, Vol. 82, no. 2, pp. 54–7.
Orton, H.D. (1981) *Ward Teaching Climate*, Royal College of Nursing, London.
Pickering, M. and Fox, P. (1987) The ward manager, *Health Care Management*, Vol. 2, no. 3, pp. 23–6.
Runciman, P. (1986) Holding a tiger by the tail – the ward sister and Griffiths, *Senior Nurse*, Vol. 5, no. 3, pp. 8–10.
Stapleton, M. (1982) *The Ward Sister –Another Perspective*, Royal College of Nursing, London.

Index